Comic Theaters

Comic Theaters

Studies in Performance and Audience Response

William E. Gruber

The University of Georgia Press
ATHENS AND LONDON

© 1986 by the University of Georgia Press
Athens, Georgia 30602
All rights reserved
Set in Garamond no. 3
with ITC Garamond display
The paper in this book meets the guidelines for
permanence and durability of the Committee on
Production Guidelines for Book Longevity of the
Council on Library Resources.

Printed in the United States of America
90 89 88 87 86   5 4 3 2 1

Library of Congress Cataloging in Publication Data

Gruber, William E.
    Comic theaters.

    Bibliography: p.
    Includes index.
    1. Comedy—History and criticism. 2. Theater
audiences. I. Title.
PN1922.G78 1986   792'.09'0917   85-16541
ISBN 0-8203-0829-3

For Laura and Elaine

Contents

Acknowledgments ix
Introduction 1

PART I Ancient Models 9
  1 Dramatic Illusion in Greek Old Comedy 11
  2 The Comedy of Plautus 42

PART II Renaissance Models 67
  3 Festive Comedy: *Bartholomew Fair* 71
  4 Shamming Illness and Shamming Identity: Doctors and Actors in *Le malade imaginaire* 100

PART III Modern Models 123
  5 *The Cherry Orchard:* Text Versus Performance 125
  6 Comedy, Community, and the Anonymous Audience: Dürrenmatt's *Der Besuch der alten Dame* 146

  Afterword: On Actors and Theatrical Genres 165
  Notes 169
  Works Cited 187
  Index 195

Acknowledgments

Many people helped me make this book. I thank them all; without their wisdom and kindness, I could never have written it. I am grateful to Jerry Beaty, who read and commented extensively on an early draft, and to James Flannery of Theater Emory, who offered keen theatrical criticism. Georgia Christopher, Frank Manley, and Harry Rusche offered much advice on seventeenth-century drama, and John Sitter made many helpful suggestions to clarify my ideas or improve my prose. On Greek theater I benefited from the expertise of Bella Zweig and Robert Bauslaugh, who encouraged my work and saved me from errors of interpretation or logic. I am also indebted to Thomas Postlewait and Roger Herzel for their scrupulous criticisms. Whatever errors remain are mine alone.

Two grants facilitated writing in the early stages: I received a stipend from the Emory University Research Committee in 1981, and a Faculty Development Award from Emory College in 1982. On occasion I borrow a sentence or two from my own journal articles; the editors of *Comparative Drama, Genre,* and *Helios* have kindly given permission to reprint this material.

Two debts are specially meaningful to me. I owe much to my father, William I. Gruber, who provided me with literal translations of *Epidicus* and Donatus's commentaries on Terence and who helped me with my own translations of Plautus's text. And I owe much gratitude to my wife, Nancy, and to my daughters, Elaine and Laura—more than I can ever tell.

Introduction

> There was speech in their dumbness,
> language in their very gesture.
> —1. Gentleman, *The Winter's Tale* (V.II.13–14)

I wrote this book to settle my doubts that comic theory adequately explains comic theater. I intended to present not a comprehensive theory of comedy but a sequence of essays with a common method. Broadly speaking, I have tried to read six comedies for their meaning as theater. I emphasize not only "plot" or "character" or "theme" but also the essentials of dramatic performance—watching and acting. Instead of beginning with a definition of comedy, I therefore begin with the realities of genre. The first characteristic of literature is that it is written, says Derrida; but the first characteristic of drama is that it is acted before an audience. Drama begins with seeing, and even the briefest reflection suggests that audiences do not hunger merely for credible likenesses of human beings. As I will argue throughout this book, audiences respond to the representing as well as to the representation itself. The actor's body is too obviously present as a resource to be confined wholly within the "dramatic illusion." The persona looms as a speculative limit, while the actor's material presence stubbornly resists all efforts (whether they are his—or her—own or those of spectators) to breach it. Certain modes of acting stress mutual resistance of player and role, as in transvestite or minstrel performances, but even in naturalistic representations the audience never entirely loses sight of the actor acting. The actor's behavior is a lie, a fiction validated by a reality which at the same time resists and threatens it. At this point we encounter formidable barriers—no single English word names the *Figur* visible to onlookers—but if criticism of drama is to be vital, it must somehow overcome the limitations of the printed text. Not just character but also the approach to character matters, and the actor-character alloy yields, upon analysis, evidence of the larger and more important relationships between the play and its public. I believe that we can read the central roles of dramatic texts for clues regarding these relationships. In talking about comedy, then, I examine plays for their value as expressive art, concentrating on the interaction of performer with beholder and on visual realities as well as on the verbal. Whenever possible I view plays as texts for acting, treating every word as a performed word and the script as source for histrionic strategy. Aristotelian mimetic theory alone cannot sustain such an inquiry; in addition we must consider the extent to which the performance calls the text into question.

As an example of the general implications of this matter, consider a Restoration production of Nahum Tate's *King Lear,* in which the part of Cordelia was played by the promiscuous Mrs. Barry. When, during a tense moment in Act III, Mrs. Barry/Cordelia proclaimed herself "Arm'd in my Virgin Innocence," the ensuing horse laughs from the audience halted the performance and, in the words of one spectator, turned to ridicule "the scene of generous Pity and Compassion."[1] It was apparently not a case of bad acting, nor was there anything mysterious or perverse in the spectators' laughter. Henri Bergson might explain such laughter as resulting from the "reciprocal interference of series"; an audience, according to Bergson, would in this instance "waver between the possible meaning and the real, and it is this mental see-saw between two contrary interpretations which is at first apparent in the enjoyment we derive from an equivocal situation."[2]

Such an explanation clarifies the psychology of the onlookers' outburst, but Bergson's theory has an important corollary. Mrs. Barry's audience could not possibly savor a sudden switch from persona to performer unless it had been silently assessing the relationship between the two all along. In particular, the audience must have been contemplating the actor—and not just the "character"—as a sexual object. We cannot of course specify the fantasies of the various individual members of that audience, but the anecdote accords perfectly with our knowledge of Restoration theatergoers' general interests and behavior. Restoration spectators normally "read" their actresses in terms of a "lively, even obsessive concern with . . . sexuality."³ Mrs. Barry's "unmasking" therefore did not surprise her onlookers by revealing something they had forgotten but rather underscored knowledge they already possessed and were integrating into their response to the performance.

In reading plays as scripts for acting, we are by no means restricted to existing documentations of actual performances. Sometimes performance realities may be adduced from the text itself or from its general historical context. Consider the performance of Aristophanes' *Lysistrata*, early in 411 B.C. In this instance, records are scanty. We do not even know for which festival Aristophanes wrote, whether the Lenaea or the Great Dionysia. The comedy treats the familiar Aristophanic themes of war, peace, and sex, and its ostensible goal is the equally familiar ambition of Panhellenic harmony. To bring the Peloponnesian War to an end, Lysistrata and a select group of Athenian wives decide to forswear sex until their husbands stop fighting. The men soon grow desperate, and jokes about erections are ubiquitous. As is often the case in Aristophanes, however, sexual and political matters are difficult to disentangle. Lysistrata argues at one point that Athens needs good sense, not *mochloi* ("rams" or "bolts," as for a doorway), while at the end of the comedy the women bring Spartan and Athenian males together in reconciliation, holding them by their erect phalluses.⁴

Does the fact that "Lysistrata" was a male in disguise have any bearing on the meaning of the comedy? We have every reason to think so. Though women in *Lysistrata* are nominally the play's "heroes," they do not differ from women in other Aristophanic comedies in that they are sexually shameless, much less able than men to lead chaste lives. As even the relatively high-minded Lysistrata eventually concedes, "we must fuck" (715).⁵ Humor at the expense of women is integral to the play and was unquestionably relevant for Aristophanes' patriarchal audience. From a psychodynamic standpoint, then, the actors' transvestism signifies more than unacknowledged theatrical convention. At the least it is a visual manifestation of the comedy's tendentious wit. The *representing* is at issue: the rhythm of the acting which imitates the women is doubtless aggressive, even hostile. Such a performance style is certainly of a piece with the overall performance tradition of Old Comedy, which is critical, negative, attacking. Given our present knowledge of the psychic life of fifth-century Athenians, it seems possible, then, that *Lysistrata* was more than intellectual satire or rejuvenative celebration. The comedy may also be interpreted as an elaborate affective structure for presenting and negotiating the anxieties that a patriarchal order felt about women. Here, too, the actor figures in the production of meaning. As in some modes of children's play, imitation may be an instrument for coping with fear or for expressing hostility. The male actor visibly usurps a woman's identity and social role; miming the female, he thereby declares all females superfluous while ironically paying tribute to their continuing power over his imaginative life. His transvestism is neither unseen nor pathological. Like many devices common to magic and rite, it is deliberately provocative, fascinating, talismanic. He does not persuade spectators to ignore his actual gender but uses his problematic sexuality to figure forth mysteries of human identity: *what is it that denies me what I will me to be?*

We might equally well turn from individual productions of plays to the entire stage history of a character, Shakespeare's Shylock. As everyone now agrees, Elizabethans would not have sympathized with Shylock but would have considered him essentially a humorous figure. *The Merchant of Venice* was staged twice in 1605 and was then ignored for nearly a century and a half (though an adaptation, *The Jew of Venice,* was staged frequently in the first decades of the eighteenth century, when Shylock was played by Doggett, a noted low comedian). Charles Macklin, a famous comic actor, reintroduced Shakespeare's play at Drury Lane in 1741, bringing to Shylock a "terrifying ferocity" which deeply impressed witnesses to the performance.[6] During the Romantic period, Edmund Kean made his London debut as Shylock; he played with a "terrible energy" that prompted William Hazlitt to say, "Our sympathies are much oftener with him than with his enemies."[7] Sir Henry Irving's Victorian productions also stressed Shylock's capacity for ennobled suffering, and one American production in 1893 reached its climax with Shylock's tragic suicide. Max Reinhardt in 1921 turned the play into a farce (Shylock was flat-footed and talked and laughed in an exaggerated manner). More recent interpreters have highlighted Shylock's wild swings of mood, somewhat in the manner of Macklin.

It would obviously be silly to say that audiences who applauded these subsequent productions lacked the fine sensibilities of Shakespeare's playgoers, just as it would be silly to debate whether Kean's Shylock is better than Irving's or whether Macklin's is better than Dogget's. As folklorists now cheerfully accept that there may be many Cinderellas but no Cinderella, and as physicists wait patiently for a proton to decay, so students of theater history may find themselves forced to abandon belief in the long-term stability of character. J. L. Styan has recently suggested as much, noting, "Because every new actor's personality must interact with his part, the study of stage history insists that we should no longer look for definite characterization, but rather for the spectrum of a character."[8] We should not, however, infer that there is no "right" production for a play if by "right" we mean for that play in its historical context. We should conclude that the hermeneutics of drama must not automatically presuppose a stable text, nor can the text stand as an ideal which any performance in any age must realize. As no narrative is ever independent of the occasion of its telling, so no play is ever independent of its performance. This dependence does not radically diminish the text's importance in criticism of drama. The text is still primary, but it is no longer separate from the needs of its viewers or from other contemporary forms of expression.

We now know enough about plays and their historical contexts to understand that they are neither mirrors of contemporary reality nor messages telegraphed to passive audiences. Indeed, the play's full situation—its generic context, the interests of its audience, and the manner and circumstances of its performance—all contribute to the relationship between the work and its public. Each of the six chapters in my book therefore assumes a basic cultural framework which defines the meaning of theater generally within a particular period. Each chapter then suggests ways in which comic theater in particular was significant in shaping human experience. I argue that these comedies primarily depend for meaning not on archetypal "deep structures" or on unchanging affective responses—laughter, comic catharsis, and so on—but on changing concepts of theater and on changing configurations of actor and role. The approach is qualitative; the method develops from a suggestion made by Kenneth Burke in *The Philosophy of Literary Form*. Burke asks whether certain moments in literary works might not be important because of their position: "Should we not," he asks, "attach particular significance to the situations on which the work opens and closes, and the events by which the peripety, or reversal is contrived?" Burke calls such qualitative points the "laying of the cornerstone," the "watershed moment," and the "valedictory," or "funeral wreath."[9] Rather, therefore, than search for the significance of comedy exclusively by pursuing its characters' psychologies or authors' themes, I try to identify key moments in plays (whether they are moments defined by Burke or other moments that seem equally significant) when the full gestural realm of theater within a historical period is made visible.

Chapters 1 and 2 treat classical comedies, Aristophanes' *Thesmophoriazusae* and Plautus's *Epidicus*, respectively. Chapters 3 and 4 discuss plays of the English Renaissance and French neoclassical stage, Jonson's *Bartholomew Fair* and Molière's *Le malade imaginaire*. In the final chapters I discuss two plays of the modern repertory: Chekhov's *The Cherry Orchard* and Dürrenmatt's *Der Besuch der alten Dame*. The arrangement of the material is chronological, but I do not pretend to have written a complete description of comic theater, much less the story of its development or evolution. Literary tradition, if the term has any meaning, is not a genealogy but a kaleidoscope. On the whole I have chosen to discuss works which are reasonably well known but are not always acknowledged in the canon of Western theater's dozen or so comic masterpieces. I have done so intentionally: especially when we speculate about the meaning of older theaters, we must guard against the misreadings which sometimes accompany excessive familiarity, witness *Lysistrata* (sometimes cited as proof that Aristophanes was an early feminist) or *Menaechmi* (which English chauvinists dismiss as something that Plautus merely "got" and Shakespeare greatly "improved upon").

I will frequently direct my attention to theatrical realities, actual or virtual (when the latter may be adduced from the text), hence some of my terms need brief preliminary definitions. Initial explanations lack illustrations; I ask the reader to indulge my abstraction at this point so that I can move more quickly to discussions of actual plays.

The concept of "gest" (occasionally "basic gest") is fundamental. Both terms come from Brecht: they are, respectively, *Gestus* and *Grundgestus*.[10] "Gest" proves invaluable when discussing the visual realities of drama. It may, depending on the context, refer to a simple bodily movement of an actor or to a physical relationship between two characters onstage or to a particular blocking or emblematic arrangement of characters (whether indicated by a stage direction or simply implied by the script). Or (in the case of "basic gest") it may refer to a recurring attitude characteristic of an entire play or (again, "basic gest") to the overall relationship between the play and its audience. Because all theater tends toward iconography, all theater is gestic and may be analyzed as such. Whether or not gest is *in* the text or even a property *of* it is moot. As Brecht knew, however, we need not settle this question in order to use gest as a tool to unlock the performance values of plays.[11]

I shall draw extensively on performance theory and will use the terms "acting style," "performance style," and "histrionic force." Let "acting style" and "performance style" describe, respectively, the manner of the protagonist or of the entire ensemble; these two styles may themselves be tied to gest. Insofar as a dramatic text is always readable in terms of its basic gest, it is readable for acting or performance styles. Let histrionic force, in contrast, refer to an affective structure; "the whole felt appeal of the plays as acted."[12] Because the meaning of a play remains latent until it is actually embodied by actors before an audience, this term proves useful to examine printed texts for meanings communicable only in performance. Clearly, "histrionic force" differs from "histrionic sensibility" (or "mimetic sensibility"), which is a fascinating but poorly understood capability that is possessed by animals as well as by humans and is therefore of little practical use in discussing the meaning of plays.

I occasionally rely on "reader response" criticism, or *Rezeptionstheorie,* insofar as it applies to spectators' experience of dramatic performance. My audience is not a Platonic ideal, although I read texts as virtual productions before virtual audiences. This activity is not as ethereal as it might first seem; if we can imagine a character from a text, we can imagine an actor playing that character in a specific historic period.[13] I also borrow terms frequently from Erving Goffman's *Frame Analysis.* I assume that the meanings of events in the theater—like the meanings of events in everyday life—are governed by certain organizing principles, primary "frames." Many of these frames are neither fixed for all times nor found in all societies. Especially in the theater the frames themselves are often at issue. Imitation, as Jean Piaget has unquestionably established, is scarcely "child's play," and the theater, traditionally, is scarcely a "safe" place. The playhouse defines a field of shifting interests and values. The play, in turn, must be considered in the context of "keys" (transformations of experience from one realm to another), "brackets" (acknowledged boundaries of experience), the "person-role formula" (a continuum rather than a settled fact), "fabrications" (which falsify some part of the world), and "scriptings" (which endow apparently spontaneous activity with the quality of theater). This last concept is especially important. As I hope to show in the course of my book, spectators' roles are sometimes "scripted" as carefully as the roles of the characters.[14]

Finally, we must consider a specific question: what do theater audiences actually see? For the sake of fluency, I find it convenient to refer to stage beings by their fictional names only, as is common practice in literary criticism. Thus I discuss Dicaeopolis, Adam Overdo, Claire Zachanassian, and so on. The reader should not conclude that I regard the playwrights' creations as real people or as realistic imitations of real people. On the contrary: my discussion centers normally on the actor/character, the Figur actually visible to onlookers.[15] I describe the significance of that Figur (and that of his or her performance) and on that basis build an interpretation of representative comic theaters.

PART I
Ancient Models

1 Dramatic Illusion in Greek Old Comedy

DEMOSTHENES: Would you I told the story to the audience?
NICIAS: Not a bad plan; but let us ask them first
To show us plainly by their looks and cheer
If they take pleasure in our words and acts.
—*The Knights*, 36–39

The comedies of Aristophanes are rich in moments when actors and onlookers become fully conscious of their interdependence.[1] This recurring image of seers and seen is the starting point of my discussion. No comedy of Aristophanes simply ridicules myth or contemporary life. Still less are his protagonists consistent representations of real or fictional people. Aristophanes reveals an abiding interest in *good* theater, which he often shows as arising from an ironic awareness of the bounds of mimesis. Spectators of Old Comedy are frequently challenged to recognize their own responsibilities as a thinking audience, and such self-conscious moments disclose the broadly educative ends of Aristophanic comic theater. However self-serving, protagonists' fantasies always address broad communal needs. Similarly, spectators' pleasures are always integrated with extraordinary subtlety into the playwright's ethical design. In emphasizing that the theater is a moral institution, Aristophanes certainly made no objection to explicit moralizing—the plays abound with his opinions on a multitude of subjects ranging from military strategy to newfangled copper coins. But merely to enumerate the specific comments that Aristophanes makes on contemporary Athenian life would be to cheapen his dual role as satirist and teacher. Theater's general importance within the social and psychological life of fifth-century Athens indicates that audiences expected their plays to provide more than entertainment or formal instruction. If Athenians indeed used the theater to put their house in order, we may profitably study both the drama and its reception by the spectator. In this task, because of its explicit concern with the actor/audience relationship, Aristophanic comedy proves an ideal point of departure.

In discussing Old Comedy as a cultural phenomenon, we are handicapped by the relatively small number of extant plays. Of the many comedies performed from 486 B.C., when comedies were first sanctioned as part of Athenian dramatic festivals, to 404 B.C., when as a result of the changed political climate Old Comedy ceased to exist, there remain only nine complete plays, all written by Aristophanes. By most accounts Aristophanes was the greatest of the writers of Old Comedy, but his theater cannot have been unique. The considerable number of fragments from the plays of his contemporaries reveal no fundamental differences between their art and his. Furthermore, there is some evidence that genres in fifth-century Athens embody conceptual values of long standing and therefore reflect clear and mutually exclusive categories for drama.[2] The relationship between comedy and tragedy during this period is far too complex to be summarized neatly, but we may safely assume that playwrights shared with their audiences specific generic understandings. Individual (and seemingly minor) variations had far greater meaning than we might at first suppose. The frequency with which Aristophanes criticizes the tactics of other comic playwrights, for example, and then practices what he has just condemned (for example, in the opening section of *Frogs*) suggests first that the poet would employ any available tactic to convince his spectators that his play was the best and second that familiar "redundancies" of genre actively facilitated communication between stage and audience by providing a context for innovating uniqueness.[3]

Moreover, comic plays, like tragic plays, were performed only during dramatic competitions, the participants being selected by a panel of judges and the winners named by general audience acclamation. The combination of genre and regulated competition must have exercised a conservative influence on playwrights (I do not mean "conservative" in a negative sense), allowing for innovation but tending to discourage experimentalism or aesthetic revolution for their own sakes. It seems probable, therefore, that Aristophanes' comedies—however often the poet liked to boast of his own distinctive superiority—were representative of Old Comedy generally.

Most of Aristophanes' comedies follow the same general plot. The play opens with one or more citizens discussing a specific contemporary problem, usually one related to the Peloponnesian War. This problem is solved by the protagonist's invention of an elaborate or fantastic scheme—a trip to Olympus, a sex strike, a separate peace—which is promptly carried out. Normally the hero encounters only token opposition, his triumph occurring roughly midway through the play. This victory is followed by the *parabasis*, a sequence of lyrics in which the Chorus debates freely a great variety of topical subjects. After the parabasis, the hero returns to the stage, and the play concludes with a sequence of loosely connected satiric or celebratory incidents. Most scenes, incidentally, are expressly obscene.

Several theories have been offered to account for this remarkable theater. Because Aristophanes cares so little about maintaining the "dramatic illusion," his comedies were for long considered nascent drama, and his achievement as a playwright was measured by his (apparently) increasing ability to write plays with continuous plots. When the Cambridge Anthropologists at the turn of the century discovered models for dramatic action in primitive seasonal fertility rites, Aristophanes lost even more credit as a maker of plots but won for Old Comedy the status of an archetype. According to F. M. Cornford, the most influential member of the Cambridge school, the plays' patchwork structure was said to effect a ritual "carrying out of death."[4] Such interpretations of Old Comedy have been revised considerably over the years, and most scholars now agree that no theater—certainly no theater as sophisticated as that of Aristophanes—carries meanings identical to those of its ritual analogues.[5]

Especially in periods of religious ferment, existing ritual

values may be either affirmed or challenged when they are incorporated into histrionic performances, so that the play not simply perpetuates or fossilizes the rituals but also provides a conceptual frame for thinking about them.[6] My own view of Old Comedy follows recent studies in the anthropology of play.[7] Instead of examining Aristophanes' comedies for mythic content, or as mirrors of the status quo, we can study them for their capacity to explore problematic areas of social process or to involve spectators in oblique assimilative or aggressive mimetic strategies. Particularly in the three "women on top" plays (*Lysistrata, Thesmophoriazusae,* and *Ecclesiazusae*), the play frame allowed Aristophanes to explore deep-seated fantasies and fears in such a way that Athenians could draw both pleasure and moral instruction from the performance of comedy.

Aristophanes' mimetic strategy typically combines representation with assimilation. Consider a scene from *The Acharnians,* Aristophanes' earliest extant drama. The protagonist, a foul-mouthed, middle-aged Athenian named Dicaeopolis, is preparing to debate with the members of the play's chorus (the Acharnians of the title). The debate concerns the legitimacy of the Peloponnesian War; just before the contest begins, Dicaeopolis seeks help from Euripides, from whose tragedies he wants to borrow a number of items. He first requests the costume which belonged to Telephus, the hero of Euripides' tragedy of the same name. Receiving the costume, Dicaeopolis holds it up to inspect it:

    DI. (*Holding up the tattered garment against the light*)
          Lord Zeus, whose eyes can pierce through everywhere,
          Let me be dressed the loathliest way I can.
          Euripides, you have freely given the rags,
          Now give, I pray you, what pertains to these,
          The Mysian cap to set upon my head.
          For I've to-day to act a beggar's part,
          To be myself, yet not to seem myself;
          The audience there will know me who I am,
          Whilst all the Chorus stand like idiots by,
          The while I fillip them with cunning words.
    EUR. Take it; you subtly plan ingenious schemes.

DI. To thee, good luck; to Telephus—what I wish him!
Yah! why I'm full of cunning words already.
But now, methinks, I need a beggar's staff.
EUR. Take this, and get thee from the marble halls.
DI. O Soul, thou seest me from the mansion thrust,
Still wanting many a boon. Now in thy prayer
Be close and instant. Give, Euripides,
A little basket with a hole burnt through it.
EUR. What need you, hapless one, of this poor wicker?
DI. No need perchance; but O I want it so.
EUR. Know that you're wearisome, and get you gone.
DI. Alas! Heaven bless you, as it blessed your mother.
EUR. Leave me in peace.
DI. Just one thing more, but one,
A little tankard with a broken rim.
EUR. Here. Now be off. You trouble us; begone.
DI. You know not yet what ill you do yourself.
Sweet, dear Euripides, but one thing more,
Give me a little pitcher, plugged with sponge.
EUR. Fellow, you're taking the whole tragedy.
Here, take it and begone.
DI. I'm going now.
And yet! there's one thing more, which if I get not
I'm ruined. Sweetest, best Euripides,
With this I'll go, and never come again;
Give me some withered leaves to fill my basket.
EUR. You'll slay me! Here! My plays are disappearing.
DI. Enough! I go. Too troublesome by far
Am I, not witting that the chieftains hate me!
Good heavens! I'm ruined. I had clean forgotten
The thing whereon my whole success depends.
My own Euripides, my best and sweetest,
Perdition seize me if I ask aught else
Save this one thing, this only, only this,
Give me some chervil, borrowing from your mother.
EUR. The man insults us. Shut the palace up.
DI. O Soul, without our chervil we must go.
Knowest thou the perilous strife thou hast to strive,
Speaking in favour of Laconian men?
On, on, my Soul! Here is the line. How? What?
Swallow Euripides, and yet not budge?
Oh, good! Advance, O long-enduring heart,

16 Ancient Models

> Go thither, lay thine head upon the block,
> And say whatever to thyself seems good.
> Take courage! Forward! March! O well done, heart!
>
> [435–88]

Following these preliminaries, Dicaeopolis begs the audience's indulgence to speak of contemporary issues, promising to tell them "startling things but true" (501). Such direct address to spectators did not exist in tragedy.[8] Dicaeopolis reminds his audience of the privileged context of his remarks: the context of his speech is not illusory (that is, it is not an image of "real life") but theatrical. Dicaeopolis stresses the specific festival and histrionic contexts of his remarks, contexts which give him more freedom than is normally possible:

> Nor now can Cleon slander me because,
> With strangers present, I defame the State.
> 'Tis the Lenaea, and we're all alone.
>
> [502–4]

Dicaeopolis then speaks at length against current Athenian policies of state, denouncing especially a recent decision to exclude Megarians from the market and harbor. His speech ends with a quotation from *Telephus,* at which point internal scuffling breaks out among the chorus. Meanwhile, Lamachus, a well-known Athenian military commander, has come onstage to defend contemporary policy. Dicaeopolis and Lamachus argue vigorously, then exit separately, and the scene ends when the chorus summarily awards the victory in the debate to Dicaeopolis. Then, turning toward the audience, the chorus begins the parabasis:

> The man has the best of the wordy debate,
>   and the hearts of the people is winning
> To his plea for the truce. Now doff we our robes,
>   our own anapaestics beginning.
>
> [626–27]

This striking piece of theater can be interpreted as

> Didactic: a witty preparation for the parabasis, the serious "teaching brief" on Athenian policy
> Therapeutic: a restorative inversion of everyday structures of authority

Mythic: the combat between *eiron* and *alazon*
Historical: a mirror of contemporary life
Autobiographical: an insight into Aristophanes' own
 personality and interests. The playwright satirized
 Euripides far more often than any other tragedian and
 engaged in a running feud with Cleon
Aesthetic: "paratragedy" is a dramatic form distinct from
 either parody or burlesque.[9]

This list suggests some of the many possible sources and motives which contribute to Aristophanes' theater. However clearly these structures are visible in Aristophanic comedy, ultimately they work together as components of a unique actor-audience configuration. This configuration fulfills a specific gest, one which is emblematic of contemporary social and psychological realities. Neither catharsis nor consistent identification with the persona seems to be the main end of such theater. The numerous direct addresses to spectators prove this point. Nor is Aristophanes concerned objectively to teach his audience certain practical truths. The temptation to participate in Dicaeopolis's obscene attack on Euripides and Cleon is too great to resist. Of course the poet hopes spectators will heed his advice, but the educative value of the comedy derives primarily from its investigative (as opposed to merely representational) dramaturgy. The stage and the actor do not simply demonstrate the comical disorder of the natural world. Instead the played word is often contradicted by an emphasis on the act of playing. The "story" unreels in a contradictory manner, therefore, as Dicaeopolis leads spectators to involve themselves in the fiction at the same time that he stresses the assimilative difficulties of such empathic participation.

Such acting makes two kinds of demands on performers, especially on the actor who plays Dicaeopolis. He must play Dicaeopolis *and* comment by gesture or word on the difficulties of what he is engaged in doing. The comedy builds toward bold visual effects, and Dicaeopolis mingles defensiveness with aggression. He plays dress-up, festooning himself with bits of Euripides' actors' hand-me-downs, donning clothes and trinkets as five-year-olds might don Mommy's hats and jewelry.

Considered from the viewpoint of the audience, Dicaeopolis's actions are clearly funny—as, indeed, children's play can be funny to adults who watch it. But unlike most child's play, that of Dicaeopolis is markedly self-conscious, strategically significant for onlookers. It contains a critical awareness out of keeping with the persona's aggressive satire of Euripides. The behavior of Euripides seems uniform or subdued in contrast to that of Dicaeopolis, which is clearly manic. His gaiety is at times extravagant, even forced. Diceopolis is not playing a consistent role but is testing modes of approach to it. The taking off and putting on of character make visible what is normally hidden from spectators, namely, the spectrum of emotions and partial identifications that combine to produce the person-role structure. The effect partly discredits the theatrical frame and produces a basic dilemma for spectators, who cannot establish a clear formula for assessing the actor and his role.

Dicaeopolis's actions are not consistently anchored. They do not remain completely within the "dramatic illusion" but retain an essential flexibility of application. As David Bain suggests of such a playing style, "the transition from audience address to action involving the actors can be as swift as the poet wishes and such transitions may be bewilderingly frequent."[10] Such an acting style would not be possible in a strictly mimetic representation, when spectators consistently laugh at one figure lampooning another. Identification between onlooker and "character" indeed takes place, just as it does between actor and role. But just as the actor never consistently merges with his role, so spectators never yield fully to the fiction. To "identify" with Dicaeopolis in this scene, then, is not merely to dump some surplus hostilities we might feel with respect to institutions or authorities. In this case the poet does not celebrate heroic individualism or temporarily tolerate disorder. Rather the actor exploits his privileged status as a character, at the same time visibly testing the role's ambivalence and limitations. Dicaeopolis is not a character in the modern and realistic sense of the term, for the text indicates that the actor is not always "in character." We have the impression that Aristophanes' protagonist is a collection of parts—an open force field or a potential for transformation which is capable of absorbing anything, whether tragic role or sprig of chervil, that happens to come near enough.

We can now glimpse the theatrical context in which the Aristophanic hero is presented. The apparent blurring of boundaries between stage and world is not an excrescence; it is integral to the performance, a kind of critical method. (It is significant, in this regard, that one of Aristophanes' comedies provides the occasion for the first technical use of the term "mimesis.")[11] Acting—specifically, the actor's assimilation of his role—is a meaningful component of the comedy. Nor is this assimilation ever fully completed so that it defines a seamless relationship between performer and persona. It is as if the actor were forced to check his own progress within the role continually so as not to overreach certain limits of identification or involvement. By means of this process there is room for spectators, too, to experience a sequence of multiple identifications which facilitate an enlargement or an elaboration of their own individual selves. Differing modes of mimesis here engage one another, and together they address both educative and developmental needs on the part of the onlookers. Of course spectators are interested in the story and want to learn whether "Dicaeopolis" will succeed with his ambitions to end the war. Naturally, too, they take pleasure in identifying with the hero's transgressions or victories. But also important for their own responses to the play are the dramatized conflicts and tensions that develop between the actor and his part. These define a cognitive frame essential to the meaning of the comedy. By following the protagonist through his own "working through" to the role, the audience avoids catharsis and turns the comedy into a learning play of considerable contemporary significance.

Because it lacks obvious political relevance, *Thesmophoriazusae* has long been considered one of Aristophanes' less significant comedies.[12] In fact it is arguably one of the playwright's most important works, possibly the central one: as Froma Zeitlin recently argued, *Thesmophoriazusae*

> is located at the intersection of a number of relations: between male and female; between tragedy and comedy; between theater (tragedy and comedy) and festival (ritual and myth); between festival (the Thesmophoria) and festival (the

Dionysiac, which provides the occasion for its performance and determines its comic essence); and finally, between bounded forms (myth, ritual, and drama) and the more fluid "realities" of everyday life. All these relations are unstable and reversible; they cross boundaries and invade each others' territories, erase and reinstate hierarchical distances, ironically reflecting upon each other and themselves.[13]

In *Thesmophoriazusae,* wit and flippancy mask a provocative fusion of role playing and transvestism. Aristophanes compounds his comedy of unusually diverse materials: from the theater, he takes the formal opposition between tragedy and Old Comedy; from contemporary Athenian psychic life—hints of which we find in the growing influence of cults, Orphism, magic rites, and various mysteries—he draws on an emotional climate characterized by sudden morbid disturbances or passing epidemics of communal delirium,[14] and from both theater and society he derives the provocative but ambiguous vocabulary associated with seeing, especially *prurient* seeing, that is the play's particular obsession. Like Aristophanes' other comedies, *Thesmophoriazusae* is closely tied to images of actors and audiences and plays within plays. But here that image proliferates as never before. The play contains few scenes that are not overt arrangements of actors and onlookers. *Thesmophoriazusae* is Aristophanes' most visual comedy both in its vocabulary and in its preoccupation with characters who spy on one another. The key terms are *watching* and *pretending,* and the action of the play—endless disguisings, undressings, spying and peeking—constitutes an *examen* of theater. Of course all of it is expressly funny, but the play does not simply poke fun at specific examples of Athenian folly. By examining key gestural moments in the comedy, we can learn more about the social matrix of Old Comedy and the psychology of the framing principles which it employs.

The heroes of the comedy are Euripides and Mnesilochus, a tragic playwright and his kinsman: a person who writes roles and a person (eventually) who plays them. Euripides of course has his real life counterpart, while Mnesilochus, the protagonist, is invented. If the main roles of the comedy thus conjoin fiction and reality, the plot, in turn, images a teasing collection of diminishing fictions.

Each fiction successively contains a lesser fiction, all of which center on various actual plays by Euripides. Thus at the inmost level of Aristophanes' comedy is a paradox: Euripides, as laminated actor/character, both did not and did write the tragedies whose scenes and characters are lampooned in *Thesmophoriazusae.*

The tragedian and his works, then, function both as satiric butts and as the actual dynamic of the comedy. Most events take place at the site of a women's festival. As was his custom, Aristophanes named the play for the chorus, in this case, the women celebrants of the Thesmophoria. The plot develops as follows: Euripides, fearing that the Athenian women are going to punish him for slandering them repeatedly in his tragedies, persuades his kinsman to dress as a woman in order to spy on the ladies' meeting and discover their intentions. Euripides' plan is wonderfully ingenious, but Mnesilochus cannot bring it off. In the first place, when Mnesilochus arrives at the festival he cannot refrain from making insulting remarks about women, and so he immediately attracts suspicion. His masquerade is further threatened when Cleisthenes, an effeminate transvestite, comes to tell the ladies that their celebration is being monitored by a "horrid, treacherous spy" (587). Hearing this news, Mnesilochus understands that he is in peril and attempts to flee, but the ladies catch him sneaking off and question him to establish his identity. For a short time Mnesilochus concocts answers which are acceptable to his interrogators. Eventually, however, he is exposed because of his ignorance of women's argot for the "potties" which decorum required at certain public gatherings.[15] Mnesilochus is then captured and imprisoned, and for most of the rest of the play Euripides labors mightily (albeit futilely) to free his accomplice. Mnesilochus, meantime, is threatened with torture and worse, a crisis which prompts Euripides to see whether any of the maneuvers which once worked to rescue his fictional heroes will work successfully in "real life." Of course they do not; and for some 300 lines the audience sees just how inadequate Euripides is as a maker of plots. Specifically, his *Palamede, Helen,* and *Andromeda* are parodied.

However laughable these events prove in the theater, they are not without tension or ambiguity.[16] For that matter, that they *are* laughable testifies to spectators' anxieties about them. The play frames uneasily both the benefits and hazards of role play, specifically transvestism. There are many images of audiences and actors in *Thesmophoriazusae,* but in no case is the compulsion to see or to pretend anything nobler than self-aggrandizement or the crudest kind of voyeurism. With the exception of the magistrate and the Scythian (both minor characters), every person in *Thesmophoriazusae* shares the protagonist's androgynous state. Most of the men in the play are epicene, either by choice (Mnesilochus), or by virtue of their occupations as actors (the chorus), or because of mannerism (Agathon, a contemporary tragedian, is effeminate), or by sexual preference (Cleisthenes). In fact, when Cleisthenes enters the play just before the discovery of Mnesilochus's masquerade, he completes an entire stageful of males yearning to be female. The spectrum that is arrayed before the audience at this point is so vivid as to be emblematic of the entire comedy. Like the symbolic deployment of maleness and femaleness in the final scene of Aeschylus's *Oresteia,* the tableau of transvestism constitutes a moment of stage psychomachia.[17] From a psychological standpoint, the comedy groups itself as an extravagant emblem of a communal "reaction formation."

In parading before his audience so scandalous a collection of players, Aristophanes seems to have gone out of his way to construct the "worst possible case" for theater. The foregoing scene constitutes for a patriarchal audience the *ne plus ultra* of emulous behavior; it is like a little object lesson for spectators. Most of the males in the audience are probably thinking at some level, *"I'll* never behave like *that!"* But this collective gest is simply one of many similarly expressive moments in *Thesmophoriazusae* when Aristophanes interrupts his fantastic schemes with similar tableaus of actors acting or onlookers watching. The play opens, for example, with a mock lesson on audiences as Euripides attempts to teach Mnesilochus how to attend properly to spectacle:

EURIPIDES.   You're not to hear the things which face to face
               You're going to see.
[MNESILOCHUS].   What! Please say that again.

	I'm not to hear?
EU.	The things which you shall see.
MN.	And not to see?
EU.	The things which you shall hear.
MN.	A pleasant jest! a mighty pleasant jest!
	I'm not to hear or see at all, I see.
EU.	(*in high philosophic rhapsody*)
	To hear! to see! full different things, I ween;
	Yea verily, generically diverse.
MN.	What's "diverse"?
EU.	I will explicate my meaning.
	When Ether first was mapped and parcelled out,
	And living creatures breathed and moved in her,
	She, to give sight, implanted in their heads
	The Eye, a mimic circlet of the Sun,
	And bored the funnel of the Ear, to hear with.
MN.	DID SHE! That's why I'm not to hear or see!
	I'm very glad to get that information!
	O, what a thing it is to talk with Poets!
EU.	Much of such knowledge I shall give you.
MN.	(*involuntarily*) O!
	Then p'raps (excuse me) you will tell me how
	Not to be lame to-morrow, after this.
	[5–24]

After teasing Mnesilochus with philosophical abstractions and the pleasures of voyeurism, Euripides takes his relation over to Agathon's house. Once they are there, Mnesilochus's schooling becomes expressly theatrical, expressly sexual. Euripides shows him the playwright's dwelling and provides graphic descriptions of the tragedian's effeminacy. Then, having explained to his naive companion the sort of "man" who writes tragedies, Euripides turns Mnesilochus into an onstage spectator, drawing him to one side in order to observe the activities of Agathon's servant:

> But step aside: I see his servant coming.
> See, he has myrtles and a pan of coals
> To pray, methinks, for favourable rhymes.
>   [36–38]

When Mnesilochus and Euripides move to the stage perimeter, spectators' eyes move with them. Because of their position, the pair become a minor chorus. Euripides continues Mnesilochus's education in the theater, attempting next to teach him how to attend to a histrionic performance. But Mnesilochus proves to be a poor pupil and makes an even poorer audience. Unlike his sophisticated companion, he cannot keep quiet and constantly interrupts the servant's activities with obscene jests. He seems to associate spectating with aggression, especially sexual aggression:

> SERVANT. All people be still!
> Allow not a word from your lips to be heard,
> For the Muses are here, and are making their odes
>   In my Master's abodes.
> Let Ether be lulled, and forgetful to blow,
> And the blue sea-waves, let them cease to flow,
>   And be noiseless.
> MN.   Fudge!
> EU.   Hush, hush, if you please.
> SER. Sleep, birds of the air, with your pinions at ease;
> Sleep, beasts of the field, with entranquillized feet;
> Sleep, sleep, and be still.
> MN.   Fudge, fudge, I repeat!
>   [39–48][18]

The scene is immensely funny. Mnesilochus cannot behave like a well-mannered spectator, and spectators certainly identify with him in his role of *bomolochos,* or stock buffoon. Jeffrey Henderson notes that Mnesilochus in this scene represents "the ordinary fellow who finds himself in the company of posturing *alazon* (charlatan) figures; he mirrors the amusement and hostility of the audience, whose allegiance he wins by deflating the humbugs and exposing them obscenely."[19] Indeed, Mnesilochus cannot restrain his hostility and makes vulgar comments at the servant: *mon bineisthai* (50; a straightforward vulgarity roughly equivalent to "get fucked") and *kai laikazei* (57; a reference to pederastic fornication).[20]

What really provokes Mnesilochus's scorn, however, is the tragic poet Agathon. When the playwright is first rolled into view on the *ekkyklema,* Mnesilochus comments that he "sees" Cyrene, apparently a well-known courtesan. But, he continues, he can see "no man." Given this and earlier comments on Agathon's personality, no doubt the tragedian appears pale, fragile, and soft and sings his composition with womanish gestures and tone. Alternately taking the parts of actor and chorus in his playlet, Agathon sings for Euripides and Mnesilochus. In contrast to the servant's vacuous rhapsody, Agathon's performance is professional, and indeed—judging it solely on the worth of its lyrics—seems quite skilled.[21] Its artistic merits, however, do not greatly interest Mnesilochus; Agathon's performance only arouses lewd desires in him. Mnesilochus pokes fun at Agathon's effeminate appearance, jeering at his hair, his shoes, and—proof of his homosexuality—his "broad ass-hole" (200; *euruproktos* connotes degeneracy). At one point Mnesilochus even offers to bugger him: "Well, whenever you make satyrs, call me, and I'll get right behind you with my hard-on and make [it] with you" (157–58).[22]

Yet there is more to this scene than obscene and irreverent slapstick.[23] By turning Mnesilochus loose on Agathon, for example, Aristophanes can satirize contemporary tragedy, using the pitifully emasculated tragedian to symbolize the woeful state of Athenian dramatic art. Mnesilochus lampoons playwrights as well as transvestites: how, Aristophanes seems to be saying, can you expect great tragedy to come from men who dress like women in order to write about them? Such indeed is Agathon's theory of tragic composition:

> A poet, sir, must needs adapt his ways
> To the high thoughts which animate his soul.
> And when he sings of women, he assumes
> A woman's garb, and dons a woman's habits.
>
> [149–152]

Mnesilochus finds this method of composition downright foolish, if not absolutely perverse, and—as he later observes—Euripides and Agathon have indeed had peculiar schooling.

But the audience's direct involvement with Mnesilochus in this scene is of a different order from their involvement with him subsequently. A twist in the plot compels Mnesilochus suddenly to take on the feminine characteristics which he had recently found so funny. To help Euripides, Mnesilochus agrees to dress like a woman in order to spy on the celebrants' secret rites. If spectators earlier found pleasure in watching Mnesilochus degrade Agathon, they now surely find a related pleasure when they see him undergo a ritual transformation from male to female:

EU. Sit steady; raise your chin; don't wriggle so.
MN. (*wincing*) O tchi, tchi, tchi!
EU. There, there, it's over now.
MN. And I'm, worse luck, a Rifled Volunteer.
EU. Well, never mind; you're looking beautiful. Glance in this mirror.
MN. Well then, hand it here.
EU. What see you there?
MN. (*in disgust*) Not me, but Cleisthenes.
EU. Get up: bend forward. I've got to singe you now.
MN. O me, you'll scald me like a sucking-pig.
EU. Someone within there, bring me out a torch. Now then, stoop forward: gently; mind yourself.
MN. I'll see to that. Hey! I've caught fire there. Hey! O, water! water! neighbours, bring your buckets. Fire! Fire! I tell you; I'm on fire, I am!
EU. There, it's all right.
MN. All right, when I'm a cinder?
EU. Well, well, the worst is over; 'tis indeed. It won't pain now.
MN. Faugh, here's a smell of burning! Drat it, I'm roasted all about the stern.
EU. Nay, heed it not. I'll have it sponged directly.
MN. I'd like to catch a fellow sponging *me*.
EU. Though you begrudge your active personal aid, Yet, Agathon, you won't refuse to lend us A dress and sash: you can't deny you've got them.
AG. Take them, and welcome. I begrudge them not.
MN. What's first to do?
EU. Put on this yellow silk.

[230–53]

The parallels between *Thesmophoriazusae* and *The Bacchae* in this respect are clear and striking, all the more so since there can be no question of direct influence. Euripides' play was brought to Athens only after the poet's death, which makes the many similarities between the plays truly remarkable. Zeitlin notes, for example, that "the robing of the kinsman [Mnesilochus] on stage with articles from Agathon's wardrobe functions within the mythic plot exactly like the robing of Pentheus in the *Bacchae*,"[24] and in general Aristophanes' fictionalized version of Euripides here plays a part very similar to that of Dionysus, the character created by the real Euripides. Both characters are immensely knowledgeable in the secrets of the theater, and both are intensely aware of the conditions which surround any histrionic performance. Moreover, the psychologies of both tragedy and comedy are similar. What motivates Mnesilochus to play the female is not really his desire to help his relative; rather, like Pentheus, he has a covert ambition to witness forbidden sights and to discover alien pleasures. Not for nothing, in other words, had Agathon earlier explained to Mnesilochus the mysteries of acting like a woman. The clear implication is that Mnesilochus's previous obscene jests were a defense mechanism designed to cope with a compelling fascination.

Thus the comedy is far more daring than the tragedy in publicizing forbidden yearnings and ambivalent emotions. For one thing, in *Thesmophoriazusae* the protagonist suffers publicly for his transsexual impulses. This particular scene is an explicit tableau of anal eroticism; Mnesilochus is formally degraded, almost savagely so. He is bent over, symbolically breached with a torch and so on. Step by step Euripides transforms his kinsman from male to female. He shaves off his beard, burns away his pubic hair, and dresses him in yellow silks, snood, and hairnet. The final touches are a woman's mantle, shoes, and voice.

Significantly, at one point during this laborious and (for Mnesilochus the fiction) painful process, Euripides requests his kinsman to look in a mirror in order to contemplate his metamorphosis; Euripides commands Mnesilochus—*boulei theasthai sauton* (234)—to grasp his identity as a theatrical phenomenon, from the point of view of a spectator. Mnesilochus is not particularly pleased with his new look. More important, however, is the dual approach which the actor who plays him must here adopt. He must "take on" characteristics sufficiently feminine to amuse an audience and yet retain enough objectivity with respect to the role to enlist the spectators as his allies in his resistance to it. The psychology that the actor/character enacts parallels the series of multiple identifications experienced by Dicaeopolis. Mnesilochus sees himself from the outside just as Dicaeopolis did before his debate with the Acharnians. Here, too, what is stressed is the assimilation of actor to role. The actor stresses his difficult and even painful effort to identify with the part and so makes his overall activity readable by the public.

Thus Mnesilochus, unlike Pentheus, is not simply made into an object of fear and scapegoated. Rather the mechanism of spectators' involvement with him is considerably more complex and involves exclusive drives toward detachment and empathy. A particular end seems to be served by the clearly theatrical language. The aim is to make public the difficult process of this self-representation. The comic actor is not merely mimicking a man pretending to be a woman. He must also show his audience the entire process of becoming like one. During the introductory scenes of the comedy, Mnesilochus leads the audience to identify with his sexual aggressions against effeminate males. Then, having marshaled these aggressions, he redirects them by means of an act of imitation which conjoins fear and hostility. In doing so the protagonist carries out for Aristophanes' audience an explicit social gesture—that of the man who is hostile to women yet is passionately motivated to identify with them. Eventually, the attitude "Mnesilochus" adopts toward *his* role and *his* onstage audience parallels that which develops between the actor/character and the real audience offstage.

The process that Mnesilochus enacts is fragile. As was true of Dicaeopolis, Mnesilochus in this scene is not a closed entity—a fully rounded "character"—but a fundamentally structureless combination of longing and fear. Masculine components of identity, whether real or stage props, exist in liminal tension with feminine mannerisms and garb. The actor/character possesses two phalluses, one real and one part of the comic costume, and the female costume, in turn, has its real life counterpart in the repressed portion of the actor's psyche. Other scenes dramatize similar tensions between the role and the real. At the festival, pressed by Cleisthenes to name "her" husband, Mnesilochus the fiction struggles to imagine a suitable feminine identity:

> MN. My husband's name? my husband's?
> Why What-d'ye-call-him from Cothocidae.
> CL. Eh, what? (*Considers*)
> There was a What-d'ye-call-him once—
> MN. He's Who-d'ye-call-it's son.
> CL.   You're trifling with me.
> [619–22]

Because Mnesilochus the fiction cannot invent a real name, he fills in with "so-and-so" (*ton deina*); significantly, the phrase covers both a genuine lapse of memory and also expresses fear. The idiom, in other words, reveals an ambivalence toward the feminine identity that he has been forced to adopt. The words express both admiration and hostility, as if there were something troubling about the invented self. In this case the ambiguous relationship of "actor" and "role" again leads the audience toward a psychological process which joins distance with empathy.

Aristophanes' comedy has great significance, therefore, for its revelation of histrionic process. Like *The Bacchae*, *Thesmophoriazusae* investigates the irrefragable pull of the theater—a pull which is defined, in both tragedy and comedy, as the prurient desire to see. Yet "seeing" in neither play implies merely visual acts. In both cases the "looking impulse" is subsumed under sexuality, a sexuality very much like the dangerously confused sexuality which Plato denounced in his famous attack in *The Republic* on mimesis. "Seeing" in this sense is condemned not only because looking at certain woman's rites profanes them but also because "seeing" is in fact the prototype of identification and so of permanent psychological change. Significantly, both Pentheus and Mnesilochus are punished for his unusual "crime" (and not just for unauthorized spying or even cross-dressing). Pentheus pays for scopophilia with his life. The audience imagines him being violently torn apart by the crazed women on whom he hoped secretly to spy. And Mnesilochus, too, is subjected to prolonged public abuse. Just before he departs for the Thesmophoria, Mnesilochus implores Euripides to come to his aid if he should encounter unforeseen difficulties:

EU. And now begone, and prosper.
MN. Wait a bit.
Not till you've sworn—
EU. Sworn what?
MN. That if I get
In any scrape, you'll surely see me through.
[269–71]

Given the scandalous nature of Mnesilochus's role playing, it is hardly surprising that the attack on his female masquerade comes by way of an attack on his phallus. With the aid of Cleisthenes, the women identify the spy and question him:

CLEISTHENES. Stand up straight. Why do you shove your cock down?
FIRST WOMAN. It's crept through here, and it's a bright red color! Oh, how awful!
CLEISTHENES. Where is it?
FIRST WOMAN. It's going round to the front.
CLEISTHENES. No, it's not here.
FIRST WOMAN. It's coming back here again.
[643–46][25]

However hilarious this scene is in the theater, it carries considerable psychological weight for an audience. The clear implication is that Mnesilochus has committed a blasphemous act, and his fate at the women's hands suggests a need on the part of the audience to see him formally punished. Indeed, shortly after Mnesilochus is unmasked, Aristophanes suspends the slapstick humor in order for the chorus to deliver more or less seriously a lecture on crimes and punishment:

Now 'tis time, 'tis time, my sisters,
    round and round and round to go,
Soft, with light and airy footfall,
    creeping, peeping, high and low.
Look about in each direction,
    make a rigid, close inspection,
Lest in any hole or corner,
    other rogues escape detection.

>   Hunt with care, here and there,
> Searching, spying, poking, prying,
>   up and down, and everywhere.
>   For if once the evil-doer we can see,
>   He shall soon be a prey to our vengeance to-day,
>   And to all men a warning he shall be
>   Of the terrible fate that is sure to await
>   The guilty sin-schemer and lawless blasphemer.
>   And then he shall find that the Gods are not blind
>   To what passes below;
>   Yea, and all men shall know
>   It is best to live purely, uprightly, securely,
>   It is best to do well,
> And to practise day and night
>   what is orderly and right,
>   And in virtue and in honesty to dwell.
>   But if anyone there be who a wicked deed shall do
>   In his raving, and his raging,
>   and his madness, and his pride,
>   Every mortal soon shall see,
>   aye, and every woman too,
>   What a doom shall the guilty one betide.
>   For the wicked evil deed
>   shall be recompensed with speed,
>   The Avenger doth not tarry to begin,
>   Nor delayeth for a time,
>   but He searcheth out the crime,
>   And He punisheth the sinner in his sin.
>   [659–90]

Significantly, the chorus associates Mnesilochus's "crime" with *lussa* (madness) and with mania; the exact meaning of the passage is not clear, but as a whole it seems to implicate Mnesilochus in a madness specifically connected to a feminine side of his personality. Madness, in this case, would then constitute the inability to integrate masculine behavior successfully with the repressed longing to be female. Mnesilochus is funny because he cannot maintain the desired balance. Certainly this theme receives graphic (albeit humorous) reinforcement when, at the conclusion of the chorus's song, Mnesilochus snatches a "baby" (it later proves to be a wine flask) and runs to the altar at the center of the *orchestra*. Once there, no doubt he strikes a mock maternal pose. Using a modern psychological framework, we might describe the situation thus: the actor comes near enough to the mother image to lead an audience to identify *through* him with the female yet not so near as to deny a conspiratorial allegiance between performer and onlookers. His gesture signifies the attitude of the public; it says, "You and I are merely 'playing' with these particular fears and longings."

Many other Greek dramas deal with these themes, of course, notably the Orestes plays and certainly *The Bacchae*. But only *Thesmophoriazusae* openly dramatizes the motives for such fusions of opposites. The comedy defines the wish to merge with the female in terms of an elaborate play metaphor and so points toward an alternate method of structuring the repression or explosive madness that in contemporary tragedies accompanies the simultaneous existence of rage and love toward the same object. Mnesilochus's femininity differs from that of Pentheus also in that the latter is motivated primarily by misogyny and refuses to take part in any performance whatsoever. Even when he dresses as a Bacchant, he wants to look but not to participate. Mnesilochus likewise fears personal interaction with the women, but Aristophanes makes abundantly clear that there is a connection between the hero's eventual survival and his need to come to terms with his desire to behave like a woman. While not giving spectators a clinical account of Mnesilochus's growth and maturation, so to speak, the playwright nonetheless stresses that within the *theatron* potentially murderous guilt and ambivalence may safely be negotiated by a deliberate process involving both empathetic identification and alienation.

Critics have long noted the brilliant parody which ensues when Euripides tries to rescue his kinsman with plots from his own plays, but this sequence of actions grows naturally from the implicit terms of the psychological covenant which Mnesilochus makes with the author of his role and with his audience. After a trick borrowed from *Palamedes* fails, Mnesilochus laments:

> I've strained my eyes with watching; but my poet,
> "He cometh not." Why not? Belike he feels
> Ashamed of his old frigid *Palamede*.
> Which is the play to fetch him? O, I know;

> Which but his brand-new *Helen*? I'll be Helen.
> I've got the woman's clothes, at all events.
>
> [848–51]

Once he has entered the world of Euripides' fictions, Mnesilochus is compelled at every moment to live up to identities not of his own making. Surely it is important that most of those identities are female.[26] He spends but a few moments as Palamede, a youth put to death before Troy. But he enacts (with Critylla and Euripides) nearly 200 lines as "Helen" and more than 100 as "Andromeda." Granted, any male actor did as much when he played a female role on the Athenian stage. But here Aristophanes uses the convention of transvestite acting to frame publicly an apology and an exoneration. Mnesilochus's "punishment" is not Pentheus's death and dismemberment but their theatrical equivalent. Denied the opportunity to play "himself," he is condemned to be imprisoned within a sequence of feminine roles: first Helen, then "the fair Andromeda in chains" (1012). As his "crimes" have been actor's crimes, so to speak, his "punishment" condemns him to live his role:

> Alas! alas! O yellow silk, I hate ye!
> O, I've no hope, no hope of getting free.
>
> [945–46]

"No hope of getting free"—in full view of the audience, Mnesilochus rejects his masquerade and acknowledges openly the power of the watchers whose gaze holds him captive. In that image of the actor imprisoned within his disguise, all play, all theater, briefly ceases. As the rest of the players leave the stage,[27] Mnesilochus epitomizes not merely humiliating imprisonment within the hated and forbidden role but also the painful loss of self which his acting has brought about. And so the ironic reversal is visually complete in a frozen emblem: to imitate the woman is defined objectively as dangerous business, for the imitator risks becoming identical with the mask. This sequence of the play terminates abruptly in an emblematic image of the actor who has identified too closely with his role.

But the play does not end at this point, of course, and we must consider Mnesilochus's shame not in isolation but within the context of the remainder of the comedy. Though *Thesmophoriazusae* is replete with images that connect the experience of theater with profound inner turmoil, the play ultimately encourages its audience to see that playing the woman is as exhilarating as it is forbidden. In Euripides' tragedy (the real one), Andromeda lamented her fate to Night and was answered by Echo; accordingly, the comedy now develops a scene in which Mnesilochus's lamentations are mocked humorously by an offstage voice that hurls his words back at him. The most significant addition to Euripides' tragedy occurs when a dull-witted Scythian who has been silently guarding Mnesilochus belatedly senses that his prisoner is engaged in conversation:

> SC. O, vat does zu say?
> EC. O, vat does zu say?
> SC. I'se calls de police.
> EC. I'se calls de police.
> SC. Vat nosense is dis?
> EC. Vat nosense is dis?
> SC. Vy, vere is de voice?
> EC. Vy, vere is de voice?
> EC. (*to* Mn.) Vos id zu?
> EC. Vos id zu?
> SC. Zu'll catch id.
> EC. Zu'll catch id.
> SC. Does zu mocksh?
> EC. Does zu mocksh?
> [1082–89]

Like Mnesilochus, the Scythian is technically a bomolochos. But his belated appearance in the comedy does not add to the general festivity under some comedic principle which makes two bomolochoi more "comic" than one. The Scythian is offered to the audience ultimately as a *substitute* for Mnesilochus, a figure against whom the spectators can redirect the aggressions which until now have fallen on the protagonist. None of Euripides' fine schemes has the intended effect, for as the tragedian eventually concedes, the Scythian cannot be moved by any histrionic effort:

> Ah, what avails me? Shall I make a speech?
> His savage nature could not take it in.
>
> [1128–29]

As a matter of fact, all that this "rude barbarian" *can* take in seems to concern sex; constantly he leers at Mnesilochus, making vulgar references to anal intercourse and to his womanish appearance.[28] Yet the psychology of spectators' involvement here concerns more than their pleasure in taking part in aggressive vulgarisms. The greater their satisfaction in witnessing the ignorant blunders of the Scythian's "savage nature," especially as regards his knowledge of the game they have been playing with the protagonist, the less they desire Mnesilochus's continued humiliation. In other words, the Scythian's delayed entrance to the world of the play is precisely timed so as to allow Aristophanes' spectators to confront and to work through some of their own remaining anxieties with respect to the protagonist. If the Scythian first makes Mnesilochus into a scapegoat, eventually he is himself made into one by the onlookers' laughter.

Thus Euripides' plot making and Mnesilochus's role playing, although at first ludicrous failures, eventually prove useful. Suddenly, unexpectedly, the kinsmen escape. But Mnesilochus's "luck" in escaping is not really an inexplicable or illogical gift of Fortune. Sometimes we are cautioned that the "happy endings" of comedy do not withstand the pressure of logical examination. But by taking into account the psychology of the audience, we can see that Mnesilochus's good fortune follows naturally from the psychological wholeness of Aristophanes' comic plot. The hero first behaves conspicuously like an actor, leading spectators through an elaborate process of engagement with a female role, initially suffering *because* of that endeavor but finally winning expiation for his "crimes." Mnesilochus's recklessness in taking on a female identity establishes in the eyes of the audience a psychodynamic disequilibrium which must somehow be corrected. Spectators are finally pleased to see their hero escape the women's clutches, in other words, chiefly because they have watched him spend the last hour in chains.

It would not do to overstate the case. *Thesmophoriazusae* is comic theater, and we must not deny absolutely the communal gaiety normally associated with comedic resolutions. Nevertheless, the final choral lyric is not unequivocally jubilant. The chorus addresses the Scythian, whom it has given a set of false directions:

> Merrily, merrily, merrily on to your own confusion go.
> But we've ended our say, and we're going away,
> Like good honest women, straight home from the Play.
> And we trust that the twain-Home-givers will deign
> To bless with success our performance to-day.
>
> [1226–31]

In this *exodus* we see the alignment of chorus with audience and not the alignment of chorus with hero. Mnesilochus slinks off, presumably sadder and wiser; he is followed by Euripides, as foolish as ever (his final charge to his kinsman: "run like a hero" [1205]). The Scythian dashes about confusedly, running first in one direction and then in the other, confused by the contradictory advice of the chorus. Finally the chorus turns toward the spectators and reminds them that role playing must now end and everyone must return home. In formally dismissing the audience to reality, the chorus circumscribes the boundaries of the comedy, proclaiming the appropriate limits of theater and of histrionic metamorphosis. It is as if Aristophanes were here admitting that reality has an intractable element which cannot ever be assimilated into the actors' play and must in the end overcome it. The Scythian admits no seeming, and the violence which he would inflict upon the actor/hero cannot be defeated, cannot even be appeased, can only be avoided—and avoidance cannot be accomplished without the grace of the audience.

In *Thesmophoriazusae* Aristophanes takes something essentially unformed and fearful and, by means of an elaborate play metaphor, delimits for his audience the boundaries of Dionysian experience. The comedy might be described as an invention for transforming potentially explosive emotional combinations into the fantasies of naughty boys. Of course it is supremely funny. Nevertheless, Aristophanes does not offer his spectators easy modes of celebration or wish fulfillment. *Thesmophoriazusae* is a learning play of considerable significance, more so for its value as psychodrama than for any portable advice on policy or life. For modern readers, therefore, the comedy is of great historical interest. It serves to emphasize a truth often overlooked, that women not simply are suppressed or rendered invisible in a patriarchal society but are also an object of considerable imaginative concern. To say more is clearly speculation, but surely a comedy such as *Thesmophoriazusae* must have been vital in expressing and even redressing serious psychic imbalances in the contemporary relationship between men and women.

When we examine the capacity of theater to effect social change, the psychodynamics of the actor-audience relationship assume crucial importance. Aristophanic theater expressly implicates spectators in the role play of the protagonists, obliging them both to acknowledge the actors' presence and to live through the consequences of their play. The rhythm of Aristophanes' comic theater is innovative, explorative, full of risk—Mnesilochus must change, play a dangerous role, take command of the stage, live by his wits before a mob. His chief task onstage is to elude the clutches of the onstage audience, the chorus. Far from being a ritual "element" that identifies Aristophanes' debt to archaic predramatic structures, the chorus of Old Comedy is a supremely *theatrical* instrument that in this play as well as in others is capable of great sophistication.[29] Initially suspicious, even threatening toward the hero, the chorus of *Thesmophoriazusae* supplies the protagonist with an aggressive drive against which his performance will be measured.[30] The hero of the comedy, in turn, must try to win the chorus over to his side, a task which he accomplishes by means of an elaborate piece of histrionics. To be sure, Aristophanes' chorus offers Athenians advice on local matters. But their most important function, histrionically speaking, is to lead the actual onlookers through a developmental psychology analogous to that enacted by the protagonist, whereby the forbidden portions of the self are ultimately integrated or acknowledged rather than suppressed or compensated by way of catharsis.

Aristophanes recreates in *Thesmophoriazusae* the bare image of the dramatic performance—a solitary performer surrounded by a crowd that contemplates him with awe and suspicion. Such a pattern of basic histrionic endeavor exists in many of Aristophanes' comedies. The hostile Acharnians are won over by Dicaeopolis's histrionics as much as by his political savvy. And other plays too end with the chorus's enthusiastic approval of an actor's performance. *Wasps,* for example, culminates with the chorus's applause for the dancing Philocleon, who is dressed as a Maenad; *Birds* and *Peace* also end with choral celebrations of the hero's accomplishments as an actor. In *Thesmophoriazusae* there is an ironic inversion of this pattern, the hero being first "punished" for a "bad" performance, one that could not withstand the scrutiny of its onstage audience.

The choral parabasis, on the other hand—the direct and topical address to the spectators—functions differently in performance. Here the chorus does not sympathetically extend and define the mind of the audience but rather challenges the audience to engage the comedy. Sometimes assumed to be an "undramatic" or at least "extradramatic" remnant of an original *komos,* the parabasis is rarely discussed as a piece of theater. Indeed, it was once believed that the singing of the parabasis concluded the ancient nucleus of comedy, that nucleus thought to consist of *parados* (the choral entry), *agon* (the ritual combat), and parabasis (the breaking of the "illusion" and the obvious termination of any "play"). To this ritualistic core, so the theory went, were gradually attached short satiric skits of "feasting and reward" which had little—sometimes nothing—to do with the main action.

This interpretation has been discredited for some time;[31] I mention it only to illustrate the possible consequences when dramatic criticism ignores theatrical realities. I do not deny that Old Comedy owes heavy debts to ancient rites or that Aristophanes uses his parabases to pronounce his judgments on the problems of Athens. But one component of the parabasis is explicable only in terms of basic histrionic awareness. Turning to face the assembled spectators and moving toward them, the chorus in its parabasis looses on the audience a quantity of outward-directed aggression. The most pointed personal satires were included in the parabasis, and spectators could never be entirely sure that their activities were sufficiently unimportant to escape Aristophanes' scorn. Tensions, therefore, must surely have been high. Yet the parabasis constitutes a more diffuse threat to the audience as well. When, in *Thesmophoriazusae*, the chorus of "women" celebrants abandons the illusion that it consists of actors obeying a script, spectators are likely to be disconcerted. The sensation is a little like discovering that the actors are leaving the stage and are headed for your lap— never a cause for rejoicing, no matter how many times we experience it. Suddenly the spectators must confront their own roles as onlookers at a histrionic performance, and (as Mnesilochus and Pentheus discovered) anonymity is no longer possible. Thus the parabasis compels the seers to acknowledge that *their* role in the theatrical event is "scripted" every bit as vigorously as that of the actors. As the chorus sings in the parabasis of *Wasps,*

> But you, ye numberless myriads, stay
> And listen the while to me.
> Beware lest the truths I am going to say
> Unheeded to earth should fall;
> For that were the part of a fool to play,
> And not your part at all.
>
> [1010–14]

Far from representing a bothersome legacy from ancient rite, the parabasis completes the basic gestural reality of Old Comedy.

In *The Actor's Freedom,* Michael Goldman proposes that "the leading role or roles of any play act out some version of a half-allowed, blasphemous, and sacred freedom characteristic of the era in which the play was written." He continues:

> A culture's leading dramatic roles reflect its attitudes to actors and acting; but even more they reflect its sense of where, outside the theater, terrific energies are likely to appear. The ambivalent energies aroused by theater-going congregate in the person of the hero, and are released by the blasphemous/sacred freedom he pursues. He is always in some sense an actor who carries his acting to an extreme and is punished for it, or threatened with punishment. In comedy, his extremism is frequently disguised or protected, the punishment displaced, dispelled, or transformed. . . . In non-comic drama, the formula is more nakedly at work.[32]

So we return to cultural realities and to historical fact. Aristophanic comedy develops only in conjunction with Attic tragedy, both theaters appearing during the reorganization of Greek mental life occasioned by the establishment of the polis and by profound changes within the psychic life of the Greek family. Polarized, Greek tragedy and comedy together form a theater of extreme ambivalence. The plays constitute an enormous and sprawling discourse of reason and madness, lust and restraint, *amathia* and *sophia*—a drama which again and again discloses explosive combinations of malignant women and emasculated men. "At the same time," as Bennett Simon observes, "it is a drama of childhood and childish fantasies . . . , and by rotating the axes of the *Bacchae* only a few degrees we can see it as a game in the nursery. It presents infantile theories of sexuality and childbirth. Is sex murder or eating? Can babies be born from a father's thigh as well as from a mother's uterus? Where is daddy in the birth? We only know what mommy does. When and where can I peek at what goes on in private? In the nighttime, in the daytime? Is it safe to look, and can one just look and not participate?"[33] Most of these child's questions are also expressly *theatrical* questions, questions occasioned by the desire to perform and also to witness a performance, to watch and to be watched. Then, as now, there is no clear way to resolve the ambiguous tensions which shape the confrontation between seer and seen, between the actor and his audience, nor is there any clear way to explain the crimes and the punishment, the source of feeling guilty for looking and being looked at. For the Athenians, the meeting of actors and audiences was scripted repeatedly with a language in which theater and sex were interchangeable metaphors. This statement applies as much to comedy as to tragedy. Hence if we are to understand finally the meaning of Aristophanes' comic theater, it and Greek tragedy must be seen not as distinct dramatic forms with separate histories and achievements but as part of the enormous and probably unique changes then occurring within Athenian culture. We cannot in the end divorce the meaning of Aristophanic comedy from that of the tragedy with which it was contemporary: if we rotate the dramatic axes of *The Bacchae*, we discover *Thesmophoriazusae;* if we look again at the apparently harmless and laughable transvestism of Aristophanes's comedy, we see the horrible rendering of self that Pentheus suffers at the hands of the Bacchantes. In both cases we confront not comic or tragic archetypes but original dramatic configurations whose meanings depend on actual histrionic performance.

The play I will examine next is Plautus's *Epidicus,* a work which represents New Comedy and which therefore exemplifies the familiar comic form which extends from Aristophanes' *Plutus* to the writings of Oscar Wilde and T. S. Eliot. Although he has unquestionably influenced more playwrights than any other dramatist, Plautus's reputation has long suffered, first from the widespread misconception that he merely translated Greek plays into street Latin and next from the belief that Plautus's real contribution to the theater was to provide plots which subsequent dramatists could "revitalize" or "greatly deepen." In fact, we shall see that Plautine comedy for attentive audiences is plenty deep, working for Republican Romans like a kind of highly charged magic.

2 The Comedy of Plautus

> STRATIPPOCLES. Ah, I'd be willing to pay a pretty price for Epidicus's assistance now. I'll have that fellow flogged till he's irrigated and then sent to the mill, unless he gets me a hundred and sixty pounds today before the last syllable of the sum has left my lips.
> EPIDICUS. (*aside, dryly*) Saved! A pleasant promise, and one he means to keep, I trust. Here's a picnic prepared for my shoulder-blades perfectly free of charge. I'll to him.
> —Plautus, *Epidicus,* 119–26

> Torture is mentioned so often in Plautus that it may well be called an obsession—on the part of the playwright as well as of his characters.
> —Erich Segal, *Roman Laughter*

People who believe that Plautus merely translates or transmits Greek New Comedy overlook the important characteristic changes that he made to most of the plays he adopted for the Roman stage. In his important study of Plautine theater, *Plautinisches im Plautus,* Eduard Fraenkel proves that Plautus consistently and significantly amplifies, wherever possible, the role of the slave. There are exceptions to this rule of dramatic composition—*Menaechmi, Cistellaria,* and *Mercator* lack the role—but so often does Plautus make this single change that Fraenkel cites it as the playwright's most remarkable habit.[1] In order to discover why such a character kindled Plautus's imagination, it is necessary to try to read that role in the context of intrapsychic and social realities that condition its performance.

A number of literary historians believe that the role simply reflects Romans' sadistic tendencies. Because Plautus's slaves are so often threatened with cruelty and sometimes crucifixion—an obvious Roman addition to the Greek texts—Walter Chalmers suggests that Plautus was either "catering to a fondness for abuse which had been formed by the Fescennine verses and the Atellane farces" or was "pandering to the rather cruel streak in his audience which accounted for the later popularity of the bloody sports of the Amphitheatre."[2] Philippe Legrand argues that the references to flogging portray Roman slaves' degraded status.[3] And Theodore Mommsen some years ago proposed that Plautus's numerous references to punishing slaves mirrored actual policies of Cato the Elder.[4]

Cultural anthropology offers an alternate approach to representational theories of the slave. From this angle, Plautine comedy is seen as a kind of ritualized "status reversal" with powerful stabilizing or compensatory effects on its audience.[5] The comedies of Plautus, maintains Erich Segal, are topsy-turvy emblems of contemporary Roman life. The slave is a mock king, a "Lord of Misrule" whose reign is understood to be temporary, therefore conservative or cathartic. Segal writes that Plautus's characters, "by harping, as they do repeatedly, on the beatings that they intend to inflict or hope to avoid, . . . are acknowledging the everyday standards of right and wrong."[6] Anthony Caputi takes the same general view, arguing that Plautine comedy is a variety of buffo (vulgar comedy) whose sole aim in turning things upside down is to make spectators feel better about themselves and their everyday world.[7] And of course Northrop Frye's summary of the final end of New Comedy has become almost axiomatic: comedy enacts "an individual release which is also a social reconciliation."[8]

I propose to consider Plautine comedy from a different viewpoint, as a problem in acting. Suppose we were to study a typical comedy for its value as a dramatic script, in the manner of an actor who wished to learn it. The text poses an immediate problem for an actor trained in realistic portraiture: the most important role belongs to the slave, but we cannot approach that role by studying what it was like to be a slave in Rome in the second century B.C.

As George Duckworth observed some years ago, the lives of Plautus's slaves have "little relation to reality."[9] There are additional problems with the representational method: what identity, for example, is one to represent? From the point of view of the enslaving culture, slaves initially have none. The contrast between this role and the others in the drama is striking. Plautus sets before audiences a complex Figur whose "identity" is not really determined by the normal forces and institutions—family, politics, and religion—that cultures use to authenticate their members. Aristotle wrote that comedy dealt with "characters of a lower type," but slaves do not occupy the lowest possible status *within* a social hierarchy. Instead they are excluded from any such hierarchy. Their existence, therefore, is based on a paradox: physically "inside" the culture, they dwell by symbolic definition outside it. Hence the curious *facelessness* of their presence: they resemble Ralph Ellison's "invisible" man, who could not be seen because people refused to see him. And it is surely significant that Plautus compels his audience repeatedly to look at a class of beings who could not normally have been very interesting for Roman citizens to look at—if, indeed, they were ever "seen" at all.

George Orwell, in "Marrakech," illustrates such dehumanizing perception. In this essay Orwell is trying to characterize Europeans' lack of ability to grasp imaginatively the suffering of Moroccan peasants:

> But what is strange about these people is their invisibility. For several weeks, always at about the same time of day, the file of old women had hobbled past the house with their firewood, and though they had registered themselves on my eyeballs I cannot truly say that I had seen them. Firewood was passing— that was how I saw it. It was only that one day I happened to be walking behind them, and the curious up-and-down motion of a load of wood drew my attention to the human being beneath it. Then for the first time I noticed the poor old earth-coloured bodies, bodies reduced to bones and leathery skin, bent double under the crushing weight. Yet I suppose I had not been five minutes on Moroccan soil before I noticed the overloading of the donkeys and was infuriated by it. . . .

This kind of thing makes one's blood boil, whereas—on the whole—the plight of the human beings does not. I am not commenting, merely pointing to a fact. People with brown skins are next door to invisible. Anyone can be sorry for the donkey with its galled back, but it is generally owing to some kind of accident if one even notices the old woman under her load of sticks.[10]

I am not trying to make a case for Roman sympathy rather than Roman cruelty. Plautus, unlike Orwell, does not ask his audience to see the slaves so that they may come to pity them. Also, whether there were many or relatively few slaves in Rome during Plautus's lifetime may well be irrelevant to their dramatic function in Plautine comedy. It *is* relevant that Plautus chose for his protagonist a being physically in evidence but culturally invisible. The slave is impossible to see, impossible to identify, unless by some rare accident we happen to notice the "self" (or rather its potential) under the load of sticks. For Plautus, pity for the slave is not normally part of comedy, and neither is the audience's real life cruelty toward slaves the sole or even the central issue. Plautus and his audience bring to the theater the implicit understanding—a "primary framework," in Goffman's sense of the term—that the slave cannot be assigned an identity within the culture. The role is like a linguistic zero phoneme, with no expressive value. For onlookers, therefore, the role represents the absolute negative of meaningful identity. And this "negative capability," to borrow Keats's famous phrase, makes the Plautine slave endlessly fascinating for Roman audiences to look at.

Thus the histrionic force of Plautine comedy differs fundamentally from that of Aristophanes' theater. There is good evidence that the hero of *Thesmophoriazusae* leads spectators to identify specifically with a feminine side of their own psyches. But Plautine comedy involves a different psychology. There is reason to believe that identification primarily with a forbidden persona was not necessarily a given of Roman comic performances;[11] indeed, it is not clear either what "personality" was visible with which to identify or how the slave could have operated as a taboo figure. It would be more accurate instead to speak of an absurdity in the theater: an outsider is placed at the center of the representation, and the insiders are moved to the periphery of events. This maneuver constitutes an important psychological step. It does not simply pit "everyday" society against its forbidden negation but also underscores a conceptual inadequacy in the entire everyday/holiday nexus. Its unique function is to manifest a magical discrepancy which Aristotelian concepts of mimesis cannot fully express. "Identity" and its absence are visually combined in the Figur of the actor/character, as if the process of identification—forming identities—itself were the problem being addressed.

We are sometimes tempted to disparage the unvarying conventionality of Plautine comedy, especially as regards the role of the slave. But possibly this very formalism requires renewed attention. Apparently meaningless repetition may reflect Plautus's compulsion to return to what was for him and his audiences a deeply problematic subject. Following Freud, we might speculate that people who repeatedly create for themselves identical situations are attempting to master something that troubles and baffles them. Such people return to a key situation which defines their needs and their fears; their behavior, if observers notice, is termed neurotic and is read emblematically. These habits, these gestures, these patterns, we might say, are extremely meaningful; they express hidden inner tensions, and to understand them we must develop a vocabulary to decipher their symbolic code.

Cannot Plautus be read in this way? Can we not reasonably suppose that the extreme formalism of this comic theater manifests psychological tensions that the playwright and his audience were unable to express directly? Conventions speak their own language, so that Plautus's unvarying conventionality, when seen within a contemporary framework, may have concentrated spectators' attentions on problems of identity, acting, and theatricality. Plautus turns loose on his audiences a character who is strangely free and nevertheless singularly vulnerable. The slave in Roman comedy resembles the wild card in a deck, and we ought not pretend that such a being assumes his entire significance on the plane of social realism or by way of a compensatory schadenfreude.

"Epidicus": Play Within the Play

Many of Plautus's plays are better known than *Epidicus*. But familiar plays such as *Amphitruo* or *Menaechmi*, because they lack Plautus's most significant change to his Greek originals, do not accurately reflect his typical dramatic interests. *Epidicus* at least has the advantage, if we may believe a cross-reference in the *Bacchidae*, of being Plautus's own favorite. Moreover, *Epidicus* contains all of the features characteristic of Plautine theater: competition of father and son for the same woman, the reunion of families whose members have for many years been widely separated, the gulling of the older generation, and finally the sadistic treatment of the tricky slave, Epidicus, who is forever being threatened with tortures that never materialize.[12] The play offers one further advantage: in *Epidicus* the ambiguous status of the slave is exploited provocatively to an extreme, for in this comedy the slave wins his freedom. Epidicus's "punishment" is thus not only deferred but visibly abolished: "Here is a fellow who won his liberty by his craft," informs the poet who steps forward to speak the play's epilogue; "Give us your applause and fare you well" (p. 361).

The plot of *Epidicus* in every other way follows Plautus's usual custom. Events develop apparently at random as the slave reacts to the changing situations which confront him. Epidicus has cajoled his master, Periphanes, into buying a girl whom he believes to be his daughter. In fact he has not bought his daughter but has been tricked into buying a *fidicina,* or harp player, for his son, Stratippocles. Stratippocles has since been called into military service and in consequence has left the girl in the care of Epidicus. When the play opens, Epidicus has just learned that Stratippocles has returned, bringing with him his new love, whom he bought with money he borrowed from a Theban usurer. Epidicus is naturally worried that he will be punished severely for deceiving Periphanes, and Stratippocles, too, threatens to beat him unless he obtains the money necessary to redeem his latest debt.

Thus threatened with numerous punishments, Epidicus begins to invent his way out of trouble. He gulls Periphanes, telling him that his son is being hopelessly corrupted by a harp player and recommending that he save his son's honor by purchasing the girl and selling her to a rich soldier. Epidicus's plan involves a triple substitution: palming off a third girl as Stratippocles' supposed mistress, Epidicus intends to use Periphanes' money to pay off Stratippocles' debt, meanwhile selling the first girl to the soldier. This complex but workable scheme is thwarted when Stratippocles accidentally purchases Telestis, his sister. So entangled a situation cannot long remain stable, and soon Epidicus's schemes begin to come undone. In Act III the soldier correctly identifies the substitute harp player. In Act IV Philippa arrives, an Epidauran woman searching for her lost daughter, who turns out to be Telestis. In the final act, Periphanes is reunited with his entire family, all outstanding debts are paid, and Epidicus is not only forgiven by Periphanes but is also granted free legal status.

What does this comedy mean for its audience? In the first place, Plautus's audience must have been exceedingly familiar with this type of family romance. The play sets young men against their elders and nominally moves toward the creation of comedy's so-called new society. And there are the familiar platitudes: sons and fathers can exist harmoniously, the play informs viewers, and families can be reunited, if only *Fortuna* grant it.

Because of the play's many formulaic qualities, it is doubtful that spectators could have valued it for suspense of plot. Even naive onlookers would probably have known beforehand what was going to happen. Though *Epidicus* lacks an expository prologue (it is thought to be lost), Plautus normally provided explanatory plot summaries for those comedies whose action turned on recognition scenes. We may assume, therefore, that in this comedy the audience was less interested in what happened than in how it happened.[13] Specifically, spectators would focus upon the symbolic actions of Epidicus, the actor/character who is responsible for most of the events.

Modern criticism of *Epidicus* focuses either on the cathartic effects of temporary inversions of society's rules and customs or on their stabilizing ideological function. To a certain extent this focus is proper. No doubt Romans went home feeling better about themselves and their world than when the comedy began. Nevertheless, the actor who plays Epidicus does not simply lead spectators through a fictitious breaking of society's rules. In this comedy the gestural style of the protagonist rapidly becomes more fascinating than the ideal social order which his operations supposedly promulgate. That acting style puts pressure on the notion of "character" and throws the whole person-role formula into question. The approach to character which Epidicus enacts speaks louder than the formulaic plot materials. We can glimpse this in a "watershed moment" midway through Act I, when there is a momentary pause in the developing events. Thesprio (another slave) departs, and Epidicus, now alone onstage, contemplates his precarious situation:

> EP. (*looking after him*) The fellow's gone. (*meditating*) Here you are alone, my lad. You see the situation, Epidicus: unless you have some strength within you, your hour has come. Above your head is a great big tottering mass; unless you prop it up firmly, you'll not be able to keep your feet, with such mountains of misery toppling down on you. Not a decent idea have I now how to untangle myself from the tangle. I have cajoled the old man—worse luck!—into believing he was buying his own daughter; what he did buy was a music girl for his own son, a girl my master loved and consigned to me when he left. If he has brought back from the army now another wench that has won his heart, I have lost my hide. For let the old man find out he was fooled, and he will strip my dorsal regions with a stick. (*pausing*) Oh well, be on your guard, my lad. (*after a moment's thought, disgustedly*) "Oh well"— oh hell! It's no use! This head of mine is absolutely addled. You good-for-nothing, Epidicus! (*pausing*) Why should I enjoy abusing myself? (*answering in another tone*) Because you leave yourself in the lurch. What shall I do? Do you ask *me*? Why, you're the man that before this used to lend counsel to other folks. Some scheme must be found somewhere. But I must hurry up and meet my young sir and learn how matters stand. (*glancing down the street*) Ah, there he is himself! He looks glum. Paces

slowly on with his mate Chaeribulus. (*withdrawing into the doorway*) I'll step back here where I can follow their remarks at my ease.

[81–103]

Epidicus begins his speech with a comment on Thesprio's departure and concludes it by announcing Stratippocles' arrival. Technically, therefore, this speech is a "link monologue" which is said normally to make one scene seem realistically joined to another. Mimesis notwithstanding, however, one component of Epidicus's speech cannot be explained exclusively in terms of its representational value. Temporal continuity of action is indeed preserved, but the supposed realism of this scene is constantly being modified by a mode of performance manifest in several ways which refracts that realism, splitting it into two divergent components. The audience is made aware first of the conditions of the performance. To begin the scene, Epidicus says, simply, "Here you are alone, my lad" (81).[14] The actor's words define the boundary between realistic imitation of Epidicus the fiction and direct acknowledgment of the performer's actual status before an audience. Nor is this reflexive movement without design: almost simultaneously the text stresses a disjunction between Epidicus the fiction and an objective identity not fully integrated with his own personality as a fiction: "You see the situation, Epidicus: unless you have some strength within you, your hour has come" (81–82).[15] Epidicus the fiction splits into actor and onlooker, developing a monody whose tone is simultaneously "emotional and reflective";[16] correspondingly, the actor's playing syncopates the imitation, defining the representing itself as worthy of objective notice. There is no question that the audience believes it is really watching a slave squirm; rather the effect here is to make onlookers partly conscious of the actor's experience of being the slave.

As a result, there develops almost a conspiratorial acting style. It is clear that the actor partly blocks a realistic perspective on the role by drawing onlookers' attentions to his actual ontological status as performer. At one point, for example, Epidicus worries that the old man (Periphanes) will "strip my dorsal regions with a stick" (93).[17] The image surely invites the actor at this point to use his own body as a reference point, probably to the extent of gesturing specifically to the audience, maybe even with a conspiratorial wink or nod. In this context the spectators do not relish flogging Epidicus the fiction or some real life substitute. Rather the actor's effort to be the slave is made readable for an audience *as a piece of theater*. The gesture operates somewhat in the manner of an alienation effect, as Epidicus suddenly takes on a double appearance. The gesture partly contradicts the illusionism thought to be fostered by the link monologue; as such, it forms a little moment of scene building, spaced within the text as precisely as a word within a row of type.

During most of this speech, in fact, the actor is frequently caught in the act of acting, as it were, and onlookers are forced as often to take stock of the playing. The action is repeatedly frozen, repeatedly displayed iconographically. To be sure, Epidicus does not strike fully conscious tableaus in the manner, say, of the players of nineteenth-century melodrama. Neither does he comment objectively on his status, as do the players of Old Comedy. The gestures of Epidicus are fleeting, peripheral, and yet in the aggregate they are sufficient to rule out a uniformly naturalistic performance. Their overall effect is to make visible two different kinds of approaches to the part: the actor must play the role and must define also his approach to it. His acting style thus becomes descriptive as well as imitative, a disruptive behavioral style which Paul Nixon's interpolated stage directions in the Loeb Library edition capture very well: "You good-for-nothing, Epidicus! (*pausing*) Why should I enjoy abusing myself? (*answering in another tone*) Because you leave yourself in the lurch. What shall I do? Do you ask *me*? Why, you're the man that before this used to lend counsel to other folks" (96–99).

The acting style made visible to spectators combines an intense personal fear with a centripetal and sometimes psychosexual hostility (*nequam homo es, Epidicus;* "you are not even a man, Epidicus"— 96). But this inward-directed anger is neither exclusively masochistic nor an appeal to the onlookers' sadistic impulses. Actually it is the prelude to a remarkable and highly manipulative aggression by which the "identity" of the slave is captured in the process of being invented. *Epidicus* is in this respect less concerned with Aristotelian *mimesis* than with the somatic representation of intense inner conflict as a mechanism of self-invention, and the comedy finds its most concentrated expression, aptly enough, in an ultimate image of the protagonist's freedom and bondage, when Epidicus condescends to be unchained: "Loose me," he commands Periphanes, "if it is your humour" (731).[18] By first showing how fear may be combined with centripetal aggression in order to bring an exterior "role" under control, Epidicus shows how to win the power to be a spectator to one's own self and to the world. In effect he demonstrates the process whereby the theatrical frame is brought into existence. Immediately after he enacts the struggle to become "himself," Epidicus steps to one side of the stage as Stratippocles and his friend, Chaeribulus, stride into view. He eavesdrops on part of their conversation, revealing his presence only when he has established absolute mastery of the situation. Again, Nixon's imaginative stage directions provide an excellent indication of the histrionic dissociations inherent in this scene:

> EP. (*aside, dryly*) Saved! A pleasant promise, and one he means to keep, I trust. Here's a picnic prepared for my shoulder-blades perfectly free of charge. I'll to him. (*aloud, from the doorway, with mock courtliness*) To master Stratippocles returning from abroad best wishes are extended by servant Epidicus, sir.
> STR. (*looking about*) Epidicus? Where?
> EP. (*stepping out*) Present. Your safe return is—
> STR. I believe you in that as I would myself.
> EP. Have you been well, sir, to date?
> STR. In body, yes, but I've been sick at heart.
> EP. I have attended to my part of the case, sir; your commission is executed, the slave girl you yourself were for ever writing about is bought.
> STR. All your labour has been lost.
> EP. (*apparently amazed*) Lost? How?
> STR. Because I don't care about her and she doesn't suit me.
> EP. What was the point of your giving me such urgent orders and sending me letters?

STR. I loved her, then; (*languishingly*) now, now, another love
o'erhangs my heart.
EP. (*with feeling*) By Jove, it is hard when you do a man a good
turn and get no thanks for it. Here is my good turn
turned bad, all because your love has shifted.

[124–37]

In this scene Epidicus appears before his audience as a Figur who has literally created an identity which he can manipulate at will. The action contrasts Epidicus, who has learned to control his emotions, with Stratippocles, who obviously cannot. Stratippocles' public "role" as citizen does him no good, whereas the identity of Epidicus, visibly fashioned from "nothing," is shown to be highly advantageous.

We find throughout *Epidicus* this single recurring gest. It is a recurring image, a "speaking picture" which manifests the psychogenic realities of imitation as a process of character building. Epidicus's first soliloquy resembles a primitive dialogue by which an actor "shows" how to convert inchoate fears and aggressions into an objective self which he can learn to dissemble and eventually to manipulate to his advantage. So, in many other instances, Plautus constructs similar dialogues between his audience and his hero, inviting the spectators to discover and partly to identify with the conflicting forces that compel Epidicus to build a role from scratch and to maintain it against the world. Thus at the end of Act I, after Chaeribulus and Stratippocles have left the stage, Epidicus is again alone with his audience, mulling over his newly hatched plot; again we discover the characteristic union of scorn and fear:

EP. (*as they disappear*) Yes, go in; as for myself, I will now
summon the senate inside my chest to consider matters of
finance and decide who is the best party to declare war
against and get money from. (*after reflection*) Look sharp,
now, Epidicus, with such a sudden duty devolving upon
you. I tell you what, there's no chance now for you to nap
or hesitate. Forward! I'll storm the old man—my resolve
is fixed. Off, be off inside with you, Epidicus, and tell the
young master not to saunter out of the house here or cross
the old chap's path anywhere.

[158–65]

Sometimes Epidicus addresses the audience by means of an aside. These moments covertly ensure that onlookers will begin to share the protagonist's scorn for the rest of the characters. Likewise, whenever he steps to one side and monitors the onstage action, the actor leads his audience to identify with his superior perspective. It is ironic in such situations that Romans find themselves in secret complicity with a being whom, had they been polled, they would surely have found contemptible. Yet the point of the comedy is not only to permit the audience temporarily to scoff at everyday institutions and rules but also to encourage them to fathom the actorlike metamorphoses which Epidicus enacts. Most of Epidicus's asides or link monologues are framed as the efforts of an actor to work himself up to a performance; they are coachings, promptings that reveal an actor's perspective on an imminent histrionic event. Early in Act II, for example, just before Epidicus attempts to gull Periphanes, he again summons up for himself and for his audience the actor's art:

> EP. (*aside, exultantly*) By heaven, all the gods do aid, augment, and love me! Why these two old fellows themselves are showing me the way to get their money. Come now, Epidicus, come, put yourself in trim—bundle your cloak on your neck (*doing so*) and act as if you have been hunting the man all over the city. Now or never! (*steps unseen out of doorway, panting and exhausted: then aloud*) Ye immortal gods! Oh, to find Periphanes at home. I'm all tired out with looking for him through the whole city—in doctors' offices, barbers' shops, the gymnasium and forum, perfumers' stores and butchers' stalls and roundabout the banks. I'm hoarse with asking about him, I have almost collapsed in the chase.
>
> [192–200]

In this and in the previous scene, Epidicus's activities and his language are explicitly theatrical. He imagines himself taking on other identities—a legislator about to engage in debate, a military commander ready to storm the enemy—and arranges his costume for maximum effect: "Come now, Epidicus, come, put yourself in trim—bundle your cloak on your neck (*doing so*) and act as if you have been hunting the man all over the city. Now or never" (194–96).[19] But Epidicus's desire to take the part of aggressors is always modified by an accompanying desire to play victim: "I'm hoarse with asking about him, I have almost collapsed in the chase" (200). And later, even in the midst of his most aggressive scheming, he again calls spectators' attentions to his fear:

> (*gleefully*) I don't believe there is a single field in all Attica as fertile as this Periphanes of ours; why, though his chest is shut up and sealed, yet I shake the money out of it to any amount I like. (*pauses*) Gad, if the old fellow discovers it, I fear he'll make the elm switches cling to me like parasites and lick me to the bone. But the one really bothersome thing on my mind is what music girl to show Apoecides, some hired one. (*meditates*) Aha! I see my way there, too. This morning the old man told me to hire a music girl for him and bring her to the house here to play for him while he offered sacrifice. Hired she shall be, yes, and instructed beforehand how to pull the wool over his aged eyes. I'll go in and collect the cash from the old spendthrift.
>
> [306–19]

Moments such as these cannot fully be explained as additions to Epidicus's "character." They are crisis points in the comedy, even epiphanies, when audience and actor/hero openly confront one another and define fully the emotions which the comedy externalizes. We could say that Plautus wants his audience to identify with the protagonist less than he aims to create a theater audience in the first place by leading the spectators to form the theatrical frame. They must identify with Epidicus the fiction but not to the extent of yielding completely to the illusion. Spectators' tendencies to exploit the persona are constantly being checked by the conspiratorial intrusions of the actor. His gestures seem rehearsed or scripted. The moments of greatest dramatic intensity in *Epidicus* are thus extradramatic; it is significant that Plautus, who writes comedy that is otherwise representational, should override the conventions of that theater in order to build into his play moments when the protagonist interrupts his actions to comment obliquely upon them. A correspondence develops between an onstage Figur, which shows the way to live out the role of the tricky slave, and spectators, who partly set aside their normal selves in order to frame the events as play.

Lacking a fully documented account of the psychic life of Roman society during the third century B.C., we cannot absolutely prove such an assertion. Yet it is not therefore idle to speculate about such matters. It seems obvious that spectators cannot avoid being implicated somehow with Plautus's protagonist; thus there must be an answer to the questions, "*What* connects a Roman audience with this particular role? What is the medium of their identification, and what is its point?" In the case of the tricky slave, the question proves troublesome. The traditional answer has been that spectators temporarily put themselves in the place of the lawless character, experiencing his actions and emotions as their own. This position assumes, however, that the ability clearly to frame events as theater is an unvarying given of all societies—a doubtful proposition at best. There is certainly reason to emphasize the ludic basis of Roman comedy, but a careful examination of Plautus's text suggests that the audience's attitude toward theatrical performance may have been more problematic. Plautus requires his audience to take considerable emotional risks, in particular those having to do with actorlike sufferings of loss of self. Plautine comedy is ludic, but the most important rule of the game is this: because the slave is not entirely a realistic creation, his victims cannot hit back. The slave has the power greatly to change the world he inhabits, but because he comes from outside that world no one within it can make direct contact with him. His most salient quality is his otherness. Real slaves do not possess such power, and to confront one who does is to confront a monster.

The form of the Plautine hero does not follow from his preposterous familiarity but instead from his undifferentiated wildness. The comic heroes of Plautus are not anti, but simply and frankly alien, beyond rational definition, for there is an important difference between what we consider antithetical, to use a term that implies organization and meaningful form, and what is considered purely wild, by which we mean something difficult, perverse, chaotic, monstrous, unassimilable.[20] As Hayden White has noted, society's notions of wildness may vary, for they do not refer to a specific condition but instead "dictate a particular attitude governing a relationship between a lived reality and some area of problematical existence that cannot be accommodated easily to conventional conceptions of the normal or familiar."[21] That they should do so is only natural; although men at certain times have had trouble defining themselves to themselves, they could always crudely delimit their own being by negation: *whatever* I am, I am not *that*. From this point, of course, the step to satire or organized festivity is easy, and at this point we discover the correctional, or "safety valve," theories of Plautine comedy that have persisted throughout much of the history of theater criticism.

The psychic agitation produced by this mechanism, however, may itself be an end; audiences do not necessarily or inevitably go to the theater to be cured of any ailments from which they may be suffering. There is a particular kind of psychic transformation associated with the experience of Plautine comedy for which we cannot strictly account by calling it a cleansing social inversion. What is traditionally called "conservatism" in Plautine comedy proves to foster a radical accommodation to novelty. We must imagine Epidicus, at the end of his play, grinning enigmatically at his audience as the embodiment of the "new man."

I say "new man" but not "new society"—a crucial distinction. Even more emotionally efficacious for Roman theatergoers than participating in a temporary licensed aggression is the progressive experience in self-fashioning which Plautus offers them. The comedy imprints upon Roman audiences not a specific forbidden structure (the so-called Saturnalian inversion) but rather a theme of "self-fashioning." For a society profoundly suspicious of the theater, the distinction is important. Epidicus begins in fear of punishment but ends by playing at being punished, and by the brilliant maneuver involved in making him so, Plautus offers spectators the final touches they need to complete their own experience of growth and self-creation. As Mnesilochus plays with snood, hairnet, and yellow silk, Epidicus plays at bondage: "You want to tie me up?" he asks Periphanes; "Here, here are my hands! (*holding them out*) You have straps; I saw you buy them. Why so backward now? Bind me" (682–83).[22] Epidicus's tactic is superb, wholly unanticipated, and yet in retrospect the logic of the comedy drives relentlessly to this point. Only in fear does the self grow: and the moment when the self completes its growth by taking on what threatened it proclaims the full measure of the actor/character's self-mastery. Meaningfully distant now are the emotional turbulences which had earlier characterized Epidicus's behavior, for the relation between who he was and what he feared has been precisely reversed. Fears no longer enchain the self but rather bear witness to its absolute freedom.

The end of Epidicus's dissembling is finally to dissemble what once had terrified him, so that the reason why Epidicus is rewarded with a legitimate *political* identity, we might say, is that he has hunted down and assimilated the condition which denied him this identity in the first place. By playing at being a slave bound for torture, he endows his self with the very thing it has shunned, completing the self by mastering that which threatened to annihilate it. His playing, which begins as a mode of self-falsification, culminates in a reflexive self-assertion, and the audience, ultimately, is asked to applaud this complex process of growth by assimilation—and not any simplistic nay-saying to individuals in authority.

Plautine comedy offers a paradigm for the problem of how untutored audiences regard the actor and so in a very broad sense offers a model for understanding how the theater relates to the rest of reality. Identity formation, after all, is not completed at a relatively early age but applies to any stage of individual or cultural development. Without identity, without a complete self, Epidicus is compelled to exist within an intensely hostile world, and as a direct consequence of his situation, his fears drive him to act according to an idea of self which (apart from the final scene) is never clear or complete but must instead be fashioned and refashioned from moment to moment. The object of the comedy is to cause an audience to look carefully at the slave and so to address the problem of identity from an entirely new perspective. Asking Romans to look at the slave must have been a little like asking someone nowadays, "Have you ever really looked carefully at your watch?"[23] By focusing on things that are normally unseen (or "disattended") Plautus turns his spectators' eyes to the question of their own character building. They understand "identification" and "imitation" as triumphs of human growth and take that knowledge with them as they leave the Roman "playhouse."

That so many roles are like that of Epidicus, and that so many plays are like this one, suggests that the problem for Plautus and his society was chronic, not susceptible of easy resolution or indeed of ready expression. There is no meaningful identity except as it is glimpsed in the final moments of the comedy, a moment which even as it comes into fulfillment is already at the point of dissolving: *plaudite et valete*. As Epidicus plays at what he fears, he evokes for his audience the modes of psychic identification. He instructs them in the way that an actor takes on his role and so instructs them as well in the manner in which the self comes into being. To "identify" with the slave-hero in this comedy is to undergo the passage from selflessness to self. We identify not with a fixed character but with a rigorously controlled developmental process. Plautine comedy is gestic, its value ultimately educative; indeed, Epidicus leads his audience through some of the lessons nowadays taught to children: that you cannot develop a fully mature self unless the inchoate elements that constitute that self are brought under rigorous control.

Aristophanes developed his comic theater at the end of more than a century of formal dramatic tradition. He wrote for an audience who considered the theater to be vital to the life of individual and state. Plautus, on the other hand, had been dead for more than a century when Romans finally built their first permanent theater. Surely it is significant that Plautus wrote for a temporary stage, for a theater which, like the playacting of the slave-hero, had constantly to force itself upon a permanent reality which was always pressing it to extinction. Plautus holds his comic heroes at the point of maximum liminality: the comic hero is an outsider who is paradoxically inside. It is important for characters and audience to experience him, to touch him, even as they compel him to keep his distance. Plautus taunts his audience with a magical being who encourages their sadism as a means to lead them to participate in his metamorphoses.

Strictly speaking, then, we cannot speak of Plautine comedy as "cathartic" in the specifically medical sense nor even in the wider sense of an affective or scapegoat mechanism which purges the viewer of undesirable or unhealthy emotions in order to restore him to normality or "health." Neither does Plautus write comedy so that his audiences may accede to the everyday "pecking order." It *is* legitimate, however, to speak of therapy surreptitiously enacted by means of exposure to the comic performance. Epidicus cannot grapple with his fears except by acting, and as he struggles to build a playable, manipulable, effective self, so his audience progressively identifies with the difficult process of self-construction. Spectators do not simply participate in the character's aggressions, nor do they merely enjoy watching the character squirm. The one mechanism *makes possible* the other; the compensatory sadism permits spectators to advance to levels of identification they could not otherwise achieve. Plautine comedy is not therapeutic in the sense that it cures the sick, just as, by analogy, a child's play does not heal a diseased mental state. But this comedy *is* thaumaturgic in that the theatergoer comes to experience the difficult process of building an identity: and though his fears and aggressions are not cured, are not even made temporarily to disappear, they are indeed integrated into a new theatrical awareness. Ultimately, such comedy is assimilative rather than recreative or restorative.

Unless we perceive that Plautus scripts an elaborate psychological experiment in dissociation and metamorphosis between hero and audience, we are likely to find in these comedies nothing more than hand-me-down formulas for reuniting families and putting the right lovers in the right beds. Yet within this static context Plautine comedy advances steadily toward a goal, namely to train its audience in what sociologists might call "psychic mobility."[24] Within the context of a culture prejudiced against the theater, the slave provided Plautus with an ideal figure by which to define the theatrical frame. We might say Plautus found a way through the slave to teach spectators a new kind of looking. For the Romans, the actor and the slave were explicitly alien figures, and their amalgamation provides the key to the meaning of Plautine comedy. Plautus does not simply offer up the slaves to his audience's cruelties, nor do their forbidden actions secretly drain collective abscesses. Rather Plautus welds identity with its negative—the image of the actor is laid over the image of the slave, and together these represent, respectively, the maxima and minima of the self. It is an inspired short-circuit; because of it, Plautus advances the daring hypothesis that apparent selflessness could be the profoundest evidence of self.

Perhaps, from the perspective of a modern audience, these experiences are commonplace. Sociologists and psychologists all stress that humans, in order to grow, must play audience to their own acts. But Plautus wrote for an audience for whom histrionic expression was relatively alien. If his comedy therefore plays largely to untutored theatrical tastes, it nevertheless defines a way of placing the actor's art with respect to the audience that persists well into the modern period.

Modern Reductions of the Meaning of Plautine Comedy

Let me return briefly to the subject of New Comedy, that amorphous collection of plays which stretches roughly from Aristophanes' *Plutus* to Oscar Wilde's *The Importance of Being Earnest* and whose basic outlines can still be found without much difficulty in more recent stage productions as well as in some of the familiar plots of television and Hollywood. The characteristic features of this theater—lovesick men and women, deceived fathers, domestic squabbles—are well known to everyone, and I have found it convenient largely to ignore them: partly because of their familiarity but partly, too, to dispute the assumption that the comedies of Plautus are for all practical purposes interchangeable with those of scores of other playwrights. Plautus indeed writes about fathers and sons and courtesans and parasites. Yet there has been a tendency to assume that he writes *only* about these things and that his plays, and those of the other practitioners of New Comedy, are devoted exclusively to the establishment of familial harmony and to the so-called new society which the play apparently promotes. Of course these themes may be found throughout Plautus, as they may be found throughout New Comedy; however, in enumerating them we do not fully explain this particular comic theater, especially as it represents a script which was realized before a Roman audience. Thus I have studied Plautine comedy exclusively from a single perspective, concentrating on the manner in which the slave-hero engages his audience, purposely ignoring most of the other familiar features of the play.

We speak, for example, of a continuous dramatic tradition linking Menander with Plautus, Jonson, and Molière and taking the form of an elaborate and often mechanical debasing of "humorous" men, their societies, and their customs. Underlying the notion of the tradition of New Comedy is a single assumption: a Greco-Roman-Renaissance identity. This position, in turn, has corollaries: first, that comedy perennially treats familiar subjects and, second, that playwrights who create comic theater know (whether consciously or implicitly) exactly what they want to say before they write it down. Of course *Acharnians* and *Bartholomew Fair,* or *Le malade imaginaire* and New Comedy, for example, show many obvious similarities in setting and plot and character, and in later chapters I shall acknowledge these relationships. But my hypothesis remains the same: that most comic theaters are distinct and that the bases of the distinctions between them may be discovered by examining metaphors for the actor-audience relationship.

In terms of my hypothesis, there emerges from the comparison of Greek and Roman and Renaissance playwrights not an abiding comic norm which unites widely diverse authors and audiences, and which everybody more or less knows to begin with, but rather radically different answers to a general question: of what possible use are the theater and theatricality to society? I have attempted to show that we misread Plautus when we fail to appreciate the full significance of the change he made in his Greek originals. In a culture which, unlike that of the Greeks from whom he borrowed his plays, seemed exaggeratedly fearful of its own potential capacity for histrionic performance, Plautus develops a comedy which mediates these ambiguities for his audience, encouraging them to assimilate the things which they perceived to lie outside them. The slave role represents a conduit for empathic understanding. It manifests for an audience all that the concept of "identification" signifies, and if it now seems strange that Plautus wrote only one plot—and *that* a banal one—we must remember that characters such as Epidicus must have galvanized Roman audiences with charges to which latter-day audiences have grown partly insensitive.

The modern idea of Plautine comedy is that it forms a kind of social "fine tuning," that it singles out people who have grown too rigid to be socially useful and encourages them to recover some valuable common sense. Yet such readings overlook the rich and disturbing confrontation which must have flashed between the hero and his audience. From Greek Comedy, whose audiences mocked slaves *because* they were nothing—literally "outsiders"—we pass to an ambiguous contemplation of an alien nothingness which paradoxically is exalted to bear the full meaning of human identity. Specifically excluded from the visible structures of social and political organization, the slave provided Plautus and his audience with explicit proof that what was without form and organization could nevertheless be logically enclosed. Plautine comedy develops historically within the context of a general assimilation of alien cultures: during the First and Second Punic Wars particularly the Romans seem to have come into considerably increased contact with foreign cultures. They apparently did so to a greater extent during the years Plautus wrote for the stage.[25] The means by which one culture assimilates another are of course immensely complex, and full commentary on this subject belongs properly to the cultural historian. But we may note in passing that the process of assimilation involves more than vocabulary building or curiosity about foreigners' exotic ways. I merely wish to suggest, from the standpoint of my interpretation of *Epidicus,* that Plautine theater may have played a vital and possibly formative role in the Roman absorption of Greek culture. The scars, the fears, even the violence of that assimilation are perhaps difficult to detect from the modern standpoint, though we may glimpse them in Plautus's texts. As Epidicus learns to play with dangerous materials, so to speak, the comedy encourages its audience to seize and exploit the principles of the theater—selflessness, mask, displacement, assimilation, and metamorphosis.

Because Epidicus mediates for his audience certain contemporary fears of "otherness," this theater may seem to resemble that of Aristophanes very closely. But it does so in only the most general sense. Aristophanes developed an elaborate metaphor of theatrical genres which conflated comedy with forbidden seeing. Such a confrontation is absent from Plautine comic theater. These comic theaters were differently interpreted by their audiences in other crucial respects that I will briefly mention. First, Aristophanes' theater, like that of the tragic playwrights who were his contemporaries, is *festal*. At its core we therefore find the characteristic style of the Greek religious experience, which, according to Carl Kerényi, "assumes as its key situation a reciprocal, active and passive, vision, a spectacle in which men are both viewers and viewed."[26] Central to Aristophanic comedy is the concept of festal vision, a heightened form of *seeing* which embraces both the seen and the known in one grand gesture. Plautus too writes "festive" comedy—the plays were performed during special celebratory days—yet in a vastly different sense. We can imagine Roman civilization without Plautine comedy, but we cannot possibly imagine Athenian civilization without Old Comedy. The only truly festive theater, in the full religious sense of that term, in Western dramatic history is that of Athens in the fifth century B.C. Raymond Williams, in his discussion of the history of tragedy, makes a similar point, arguing that "the decisive factor is probably not [the] immediate context, in institutions, but the wider context, in beliefs."[27] The Greeks (unlike the Romans and subsequent societies) seem not to have distinguished religious experience as a special category of experience; instead they located genuine religious belief in that which was simultaneously visible and understood. Given this frame, which is, historically speaking, as unique as it was then normal, the theatron was a natural—perhaps an inevitable—consequence.

It ought to be obvious that when Romans went to the theater, they went for something else and something less. And though the spectators who gathered to watch Plautine comedy must surely have been deeply sensitive to the profound changes taking place around them, they could not possibly have found, as did the Greeks, that their actor/heroes were wondrous.[28] About Plautine theater we must remember that the emotional distance between actor and audience is perhaps greater than at any other time in the history of Western theater, the realistic proscenium arch stage and darkened auditorium of the nineteenth century notwithstanding. Though they may not have been technically disfranchised, actors at this stage in the history of the Republic seem to have been morally suspect. The hero of the plays of course exists outside the visible structures of society.[29]

Still, the blows which never fall on the actor's back may eventually transform shame into grace. Partly because they are so frequent, these threats constitute a special kind of environment for the central Figur and imbue his behavior with meaning which can be absorbed by his audience. The threats constitute a protection in two ways. Of course they chastise the persona, whose activity is rigorously segregated and repeatedly purified, but second, and more important, they compel the audience to confront the physical reality of the actor. His contradictory nature—insider/outsider, aggressor/victim, slave/hero, actor/role—overcomes the discrepancies of logical thought and so fosters growth and change.

Plautus's feeling for the theater's violence makes him and his comedy very important to subsequent generations of playwrights. Awareness of the fear and hostility that are necessary to construct and to maintain an assumed identity, a belief in the freedom of acting and in the logically absurd powers of the actor with regard to the society that surrounds him, a constant sensitivity to the potential shame of hypocrisy, and above all an awareness of the aggressive rhythms of histrionic performance—these, and not simply plot lines and literary techniques, are the theatrical essentials which Plautus offers to subsequent playwrights.

PART II
Renaissance Models

> The Elizabethan theater may thus be regarded as the
> heir of the Greek tragic theater with its ritual basis. The
> Elizabethan cosmos is still that of the great tradition,
> which the Middle Ages inherited from the city state. The
> physical stage itself is symbolic in the same way as the
> tragic stage of the Greeks; and the ritual component in
> its drama has similar deep and general meanings.
> —Francis Fergusson, *The Idea of a Theater*

> To put the matter in its simplest terms, Shakespeare and
> the other new playwrights of the time were poised
> between the traditional patterns which the theater had
> developed to represent and order life in various formal
> schemes, and a new experimentalism which led them to
> imitate life in more realistic ways and follow it wherever
> it seemed to lead.... The greater dramatists seem to
> have accepted the tension and made it the very subject
> of their drama.
> —Alvin Kernan, *The Playwright as Magician*

Thus wrote Francis Fergusson, in 1949, and Alvin Kernan, in 1979, on the relationship between medieval and Renaissance theaters. Of these differing models for theater history, that represented by Fergusson long dominated the theory of Renaissance drama. Its hypotheses were, first, that literary history obeyed natural principles of growth and development and, second, that there was within a play text a single, ideal meaning to be explicated. Opposed to this general perspective is the position associated with the "new historicism" (the term was coined by Stephen Greenblatt), a criticism which, in Greenblatt's description, "tends to ask questions about its own methodological assumptions and those of others."[1] To illustrate the differences between these two diverse critical methods, Greenblatt compares a modern reading of Shakespeare's *Richard II* with an Elizabethan response to the play. He cites J. Dover Wilson, who once declared that Shakespeare's work buttressed Tudor power because it portrayed the "sacrilegious" deposition of an anointed king. It was "incontestable," argued Wilson, "that Shakespeare and his audience regarded Bolingbroke as a usurper."[2] Yet as Greenblatt notes, Shakespeare's queen and some of her subjects thought otherwise: on the eve of the Essex uprising in 1601, someone paid the Lord Chamberlain's Men forty shillings to revive the play, a gesture that Elizabeth read instantly (and correctly) as a threat to her own position. For Elizabeth, Shakespeare's drama was hardly a historical lesson in obedience to one's monarch; in production, the play was dangerously assimilative, its applications wickedly plastic. "I am Richard II," she cried to William Lambard, the antiquary, shortly after the abortive revolt; "Know ye not that?"[3]

Greenblatt suggests that the difference between Elizabeth's and Dover Wilson's readings is partly "the difference between a conception of art that has no respect whatsoever for the integrity of the text ('I am Richard II. Know ye not that?') and one that hopes to find, through historical research, a stable core of meaning within the text, a core that unites disparate and even contradictory parts into an organic whole."[4] Elizabeth responds less to a "hymn to Tudor order" than to the occasion of the text, loosed "in open streets and houses." She fears that the public's easy familiarity with the mechanics of assassination might become manipulable by her enemies, and she responds, accordingly, "to the presence of *any* representation of deposition, whether regarded as sacrilegious or not; to the choice of this particular story at this particular time; to the place of the performance; to her own identity as it is present in the public sphere and as it fuses with the figure of the murdered king."[5]

Elizabeth is not necessarily a better reader of Shakespeare than

Dover Wilson; nevertheless, the legitimacy of her response to *Richard II* proves clearly the value of reading dramatic texts only in relation to an audience—the kind of approach advocated recently, for example, by Robert D. Hume. Hume addresses specifically Restoration and eighteenth-century drama, but his principles are equally applicable to plays of any age:

> The text has its own integrity, but considered as a play, it must be dealt with in relationship to some audience, and that audience will have its own expectations and experience to draw on. . . . Almost all new critical explicators have believed that there is *a* correct interpretation to be found and explicated. This is patently false for a great many plays, especially good plays. . . . The insistence of New Critics upon the unique rightness of particular readings has produced a chaotic jumble of contradictory interpretations which ignore the wide variety of legitimate production possibilities.[6]

Certainly Renaissance plays often celebrated or consolidated royal power. Court masques provide an obvious example, as do several Shakespearean comedies. Even *Richard II* provides its audience with a symbolic set piece on the necessity of maintaining order. In fact, the overwhelming majority of sixteenth- and seventeenth-century texts seem conservative. Given the reality of censorship, what else would we expect? But the relationship of theater to society in this period is more complicated than the familiar "mirror" metaphor first suggests. There is increasing evidence, for example, that nominal efforts to make the existing power structure seem legitimate (such as *Richard II*), far from sustaining political orthodoxy, complied with its letter, as Jonathan Dollimore suggests, only "after having destroyed its spirit."[7] Indeed, there are good reasons to assume direct connections between the collapse shortly before the English Civil War of most of the established institutions of church and state and a theater which for sixty years had presented "an increasing series of challenges to traditional authority, to king, father, church, law, family, 'nature,' and state."[8] Regarding Jacobean tragedy Dollimore argues especially that it not only "undermined religious orthodoxy" but also generated "other, equally important subversive preoccupations—namely a critique of ideology, the demystification of political and power relations and the decentring of 'man.' "⁹ Franco Moretti states the matter more bluntly: "Tragedy disentitled the absolute monarch to all ethical and rational legitimation. Having deconsecrated the king, it thus made it possible to decapitate him."[10]

The view that Tudor and Stuart tragedy was on the whole politically conservative has come under attack in recent years and has been seriously—if not wholly—discredited. But we still lack an adequate conception of the relationship of comic drama to Renaissance institutions. In the following two chapters I will explore some aspects of seventeenth-century comic theaters that hitherto have been ignored or oversimplified because of the so-called historical fallacy—namely the tendency, common in modern criticism of comedy, to interpret the meaning of the present in terms of the past. The familiar comic images of disorder and misrule and inversion are indispensable for understanding comedies of the seventeenth century, not, however, because they continue visibly a great Western "comic tradition" but because playwrights use them to image a problematic status quo. This explorative (as opposed to conservative or socializing) function for comedy is a fascinating but largely unexamined aspect of seventeenth-century theater.

It is clear, as James Feibleman long ago suggested in a critique of the logic of psychoanalysis, that examining phenomena in terms of their origins often overvalues past achievements at the expense of newer ones.[11] I must further emphasize that the embedding of older performance elements within plays is not prima facie evidence of a common or continuing core of meaning.[12] By examining two seventeenth-century comedies which use standard comic materials, we may see that characters, plots, and techniques passed on from one age to another ought not to be regarded as carrying fixed quanta of meaning. Rather the meaning of stock characters and events varies as theater audiences interpret those materials for different ends and according to different needs. As was true of Aristophanic and Plautine theaters, so here: the study of genre becomes the study of theater, which in turn becomes the study of a culture or of an age.

3 Festive Comedy: *Bartholomew Fair*

> COKES. By this good day they fight bravely! doe they not, *Numps*?
> WASPE. Yes, they lack'd but you to be their second, all this while.
>
> —Jonson, *Bartholomew Fair*

First performed at the Hope Theatre on October 31, 1614, *Bartholomew Fair* is the last of Jonson's four great comedies, and it may well be the last comic masterpiece of the English Renaissance stage. It may also be the least understood. The play has not proved easy to accommodate to Jonsonian satiric comedy and long embarrassed even Jonson's most vigorous admirers. Swinburne, for example, thought that in places the comedy was "too rank for any but a very strong digestion."[1] The play found an enthusiastic audience, however, among a generation of modern scholars who were concerned to define the value of celebration within the overall social structure. In contrast to Jonson's other major comedies, *Bartholomew Fair* was native, popular, alive with the celebratory mood of folk theater. Here apparently was a genial Jonson; for once the stern moralist seemed to write in praise of folly, not to censure it. As Thomas Greene puts it, the comedy here "leads all of its bourgeois characters out of their houses to baptise them in the tonic and muddy waters of errant humanity."[2] L. A. Beaurline too finds *Bartholomew Fair* fundamentally different from typical Jonsonian comedy in that it involves "something more distinctly playful, visceral and alive to animal existence, a life-enhancing laughter."[3]

Greene and Beaurline write from modernist perspectives on "festive" or "holiday" behavior and its meaning for a theater audience. According to this view, if *Bartholomew Fair* can be conceived in terms of a restorative "bath" or ritualized inversion, accusations that the play lacks an explicit moral center can be countered with the explanation that acting out "misrule" does not permanently disrupt society but instead revitalizes it.[4]

But saturnalian readings of *Bartholomew Fair* have not proved universally attractive. A number of critics have argued that the comedy is fundamentally satiric, either by pointing to the social criticism implicit in Jonson's realistic portraiture or by placing the work within the Lucianic tradition.[5] I will mediate between these two approaches and will consider the play in terms of the creative interaction of text, histrionic performance, and spectators' involvement.[6]

Bartholomew Fair: The Aggressions of Histrionic Performance

Though *Bartholomew Fair* was once thought formless, scholars in the twentieth century have established beyond question its artistic unity.[7] Amid all the bustle and noise, we can identify the following clearly developed story lines: John and Win-the-fight Littlewit's visit to the fair; the wooing of Dame Purecraft; the satire of the Puritan, Zeal-of-the-Land Busy; the gulling of Bartholomew Cokes, one of the comedy's most consistent fools; and the gulling of Justice Overdo.[8] The location of these actions is the great Smithfield Fair, where the fairgoers' various desires are thrown into conflict with the activities of the fair's inhabitants, chiefly Ursula (the pig woman), Knockem (a horsecourser), Nightingale (a ballad singer), Edgworth (the cutpurse), and Troubleall (a madman). As Richard Levin has shown, Jonson in this play carries to an extreme the techniques of Renaissance subplotting, binding his drama together by means of direct-contrast plots, three-level hierarchies, equivalence plots, and clown subplots.[9]

It can be argued that *Bartholomew Fair* is concerned to represent the fair itself less than to dramatize the encounter between a group of fairgoers and the fair's inhabitants. The characters consequently form two distinct groups: those who wish simply to behold the fair and those who are part of it. Thus the central action concerns a group of Londoners who initially "bracket"[10] the Smithfield Fair in a more or less conventional fashion. Whatever their individual personalities or interests, each visitor approaches the fair with a basic organizational premise—namely, the belief that organized festivity is separated temporally and spatially from everyday life. Not only personal humors but also basic human perceptions, then, are at issue in this comedy. Moreover, the error Jonson seeks to dramatize is collective: simply put, the visitors believe that the fair can be framed as "fair." They believe that its meaning for them derives from the organizational perspective they impose upon it. They try to organize it as recreation or as sport—that is, as something ontologically separate from real life.

In so framing the fair, the visitors approach it as if it were a product and they its consumers. Note that the recreational or festive frame allows for exactly this kind of unilateral exploitation. Since the visitors believe themselves to be onlookers at a spectacle, it follows that they believe themselves to be shielded from active involvement with the proceedings. They therefore assume they will be able to use their privileged status for various personal ends. And each visitor indeed tries to exploit festivity for selfish gains: Justice Overdo hopes to use it for his "discoveries," to spy unseen on criminals; Winwife and Quarlous desire not enlightenment but simply entertainment, which for them means the opportunity to enjoy watching fools; Win Littlewit wants exotic food; Edgworth wants Nightingale to perform his ballads so as to distract the attention of those whom he intends to rob; Littlewit has a spectacle of his own he intends to put on; and Zeal-of-the-Land Busy wants simply to shut all performances down.

But the relationship of the fair to real life proves to be complex and shifting. It cannot be organized meaningfully by the onlookers, whose various individual perspectives are themselves reframed or transformed. The customary relationship between holiday and everyday is ironically disturbed so as to deny the fair's visitors the exploitative opportunities they had imagined. Their organizing frames will not apply. They lose command of the experience. They flounder. Suddenly the fair begins to demand of the visitors the kind of commitments and assessments they thought belonged only to "real" life. The comedy thus becomes a kind of testing of the limits of participation and detachment involved in visual experience. Onlookers themselves, much to their surprise and chagrin, become participants, and the fair is eventually transformed into a playhouse capable of absorbing spectators without limit.

Jonson develops his psychology of audience involvement even before the comedy proper is under way. The play begins with an elaborate induction. The first person to come onstage is the stagekeeper, who enters apparently to explain to the audience that the play's performance has been temporarily delayed: *"Gentlemen,* haue a little patience, they are e'en vpon comming, instantly. He that should beginne the Play, Master *Littlewit,* the *Proctor,* has a stitch new falne in his black silk stocking; 'twill be drawn vp ere you can tell twenty. He playes one o' the *Arches,* that dwels about the *Hospitall,* and hee has a very pretty part. But for the whole *Play,* will you ha' the truth on't? (I am looking, lest the *Poet* heare me, or his man, Master *Broome,* behind the Arras) it is like to be a very conceited scuruy one, in plaine English" (Induction, 1–9).[11]

The stagekeeper's words are a marvelous compound of truth and lies. All of his words have secretly been written by Jonson, but probably the play's first spectators did not suspect that they were already watching an actor play his part. The stagekeeper's discourse is eccentric, rambling, and apologetic. It flatters the audience and reinforces the spectators' belief in their superior status as watchers of the play to come. Because of the apparent spontaneity of the stagekeeper's remarks, spectators are led to believe that they are witnesses to something which the poet and the players would have preferred them not to see. Their impression is that the performers have failed to get ready on time and that—to justify the delay and to appease the paying customers—the audience is being told the secrets of performance. The specific effect is to discredit the players. Littlewit's initial effectiveness as a credible

Festive Comedy: *Bartholomew Fair*   75

fiction, in other words, will suffer if his audience is reminded at this critical moment that the actor who will be playing him has a run in his stocking. The stagekeeper rattles on, complaining about the comedy and its author, reminding spectators that, in comparison with the glorious theater of days gone by, what they are about to see is inferior drama.

Only after some long minutes of playing time does Jonson enlighten his audience, bringing onstage a scrivener and a book holder who rebukes the stagekeeper for his folly: "Your iudgement, Rascall? for what? sweeping the *Stage?* or gathering vp the broken Apples for the beares within? Away Rogue, it's come to a fine degree in these *spectacles* when such a youth as you pretend to a iudgement" (51–54). Effectively silenced, the stagekeeper exits, whereupon the book holder directs the scrivener to read to the audience in lieu of a prologue (or so he says) a set of "Articles of Agreement" drawn up by the author of the play. These constitute a formal code of behavior agreed upon by all parties to the coming performance. The spectators are enjoined, among other things, to exercise their own individual judgments, to content themselves with contemporary theater and not yearn for bygone plays, and to refrain from scouring the play for possible allegorical meanings. Once this covenant is read, the action of *Bartholomew Fair* commences.

Partly this unusual induction serves effectively to quiet the spectators; partly, too, it reminds them of their obligations as intelligent humans. More important than that reminder, however, is the induction's intricate structure of temptation and chastisement. Given an assembly of spectators who do not have the text of the play open before them, it is impossible that they not be hoodwinked by the apparently extemporaneous ramblings of the stagekeeper. The effect is to reinforce spectators' belief in their own status as watchers, then suddenly to deny them that privilege. Jonson first tempts them to think that they can view the actors' play from a superior perspective, but in scripting a fictitious monitoring he is actually creating a trap. In the minds of the audience, the backstage becomes "bugged," open secretly (or so spectators think) to view.[12] But of course it is not, and Jonson slyly catches the complacent viewers who think they are waiting for a

Jonsonian comedy to begin. Spectators are pleased to have caught the playwright and his show with a run, as it were—whereas the truth of the matter is that in so thinking they are already playing the role written for them by the playwright's script.

For readers who care to heed it, Jonson's induction demonstrates a stage process repeated throughout *Bartholomew Fair*. By dramatizing the process by which spectators unwittingly commit themselves to a fictitious world, the comedy dramatizes the moral and psychological implications of becoming an audience to others' acts. It is an important lesson indeed: merely perceiving, we learn, is itself active involvement in the world, and objective judgment, in consequence, is never possible.

Bartholomew Fair exemplifies, then, the mishaps that occur when humans misuse their eyes. Jonson pursues two methods to dramatize the plight of the foolish bystander who cannot understand that he is deeply involved in the object of his vision. By the first method, the playwright develops a taxonomy of visual acts in his comedy; by the second, he dramatizes the magnetic pull of any performer on his audience. If the action of the comedy disrupts conventional frames on festivity, it is also powerfully centripetal. No performer is long alone; always the actor's presence causes a crowd to form and maneuvers would-be spectators into becoming participants.

The overall aim is to pack the stage with players. When Act I commences, for example, there is a lone actor on the stage, but soon the boards are crowded with others. Act II follows this same pattern, beginning with several (it is impossible to specify the exact number) players on stage and concluding with ten. Act III exaggerates and embellishes the game of appearings and disappearings (it consists of more than fifty separate exits and entrances); and during Acts IV and V so many people are on the stage simultaneously as to make it seem amazing that Jonson was able to produce his play at all, given the limited casting pools of contemporary playing companies.[13] Among other things, Jonson seems here to be experimenting in an abstract way with sheer mass, trying to assess the psychological and visual effects that can be produced by the movements of abnormally large numbers of bodies on the stage. At first the activity seems innocuous. But by the time that Northern, Puppy, and Cutting stumble belatedly and unexpectedly onto the stage midway through Act IV, the phenomenon carries troubling implications.[14]

Festivity, it seems, cannot successfully be framed. It is impossible to ascertain where the rim of the fair lies, where the claims of play leave off and yield to the claims of the everyday world. In general, this specifically theatrical pull is the source of *Bartholomew Fair*'s prodigious histrionic power. As the comedy closes, everyone who has attended the fair becomes a participant. Justice Overdo tells everyone to come to his house for supper, and Cokes urges that a group of puppet/actors be invited too. In encouraging the players to follow him home, Cokes is not merely being friendly, taking in a collection of homeless strays. In the terms of the actor-audience paradigm that Jonson here develops, Cokes is encouraging nothing less than the absolute deregulation of the theater. Whether or not Cokes's words express Jonson's opinion, and whether we ought to applaud the fact that the actors have escaped from the playhouse frame and are now headed for private homes are matters that strike at the heart of *Bartholomew Fair*.

Seeing and Being Seen: Reciprocity and Responsibility in *Bartholomew Fair*

By the end of the sixteenth century the Deuteronomic injunction against transvestism had become the central issue in a far-reaching controversy. Many people used the biblical verse as a club with which to attack every aspect of the theater, a hysterical reaction to plays and players which Jonson satirizes in *Bartholomew Fair* in the Puritan zealot Busy. Still, in the contemporary mind, the passage from Deuteronomy was no mere technicality, and it would be a serious error to place it in the same class as the absurd Sunday blue laws. The taking of female parts by boy players was not the sole issue nor even the central issue. Because transvestism conjoined the twin issues of antitheatricalism and antifeminism, it seems to have signified for Elizabethans and Jacobeans a widespread psychosexual anxiety whose implications may never fully be understood. Jonson himself was so interested in the question that in 1615 he requested the antiquary Selden to investigate the matter on his behalf.[15]

The issue had occupied his mind somewhat earlier. One effect of the fair, as Beaurline has observed, is to cause visitors to transvest themselves.[16] So contagious is this practice, in fact, that dress-up constitutes one of the activities on which the comedy is founded. In most cases the costumes have considerable satiric value. Overdo dresses as a fool in an attempt to discover "enormities." Win Littlewit and Mistress Overdo disguise themselves as whores; Quarlous dresses up as the lunatic, Troubleall, in order to obtain Justice Overdo's signature; Cokes, half-naked, is metamorphosed into the martyred Saint Bartholomew; even Littlewit's puppet characters, Hero and Leander, are transformed when their romance is vulgarized into an obscene tryst across the Thames. The climax of this communal dissembling occurs late in Act V. As the puppets put on their show, Busy frantically invokes the biblical injunction against transvestism, shouting, "Yes, and my maine argument against you, is, that you are an abomination: for the Male, among you, putteth on the apparell of the *Female,* and the *Female* of the *Male*" (V.v. 98–100). Meanwhile Troubleall (whose clothes have been stolen by Quarlous) stumbles onto the stage, naked but for Ursula's dripping pan, calling for everyone to "be vncouer'd" (V.vi.49). At which point Mistress Overdo vomits at her husband's feet.

This wholesale conversion of spectators into participants seems at first to enact on a grand scale the madness of Pentheus or the humiliation of Mnesilochus, and indeed there are many parallels between Jonson's play and Aristophanic Old Comedy in particular.[17] Overdo, like Mnesilochus, dresses like one of the holiday celebrants in order to spy on them, and like Mnesilochus, Overdo is brutalized as a consequence. But the meaning of Overdo's interaction with the celebrants turns out to be quite different from that dramatized by Aristophanes. Mnesilochus longs to close with a forbidden possibility of self; he wants to see what it is like to be the female. Overdo, however, does not want to *look* in order to identify with repressed possibilities of self. He professes only a dispassionate interest in the objects of his vision. Like the principal who installs a one-way mirror in the toilet to spy on drug transactions, Overdo wants to monitor criminal activity. He cannot effectively mete out justice, he complains, because men who are "publike persons" cannot know reality firsthand. He must depend for his information on questionable sources—informants, or stool pigeons. "Nay, what can wee know?" he laments; "wee heare with other mens eares; wee see with other mens eyes; a foolish Constable, or a sleepy Watchman, is all our information (II.i.28–31). Overdo's plan to remedy this situation befits his intellect. His disguise, he hopes, will enable him to "spare spy money" by making his own "discoueries" (II.i.40–41).

At first we may think we are hearing a simple Jonsonian satire of fools: "They may haue seene many a foole in the habite of a Iustice," Overdo remarks, "but neuer till now, a Iustice in the habit of a foole" (II.i.7–9). But there are troubling resonances to Overdo's words, specifically those in which he elaborates what he considers the chief value of his disguise. What seems to interest him most is that his disguise confers both power and invisibility. Indeed it is difficult to tell which thrills him more, the power or the invisibility, so entangled are those motives in his mind as he alternately imagines himself as God sitting in judgment or as a mere mortal spying on scenes which he normally could not see: "Here is my blacke booke, for the purpose; this the cloud that hides me: vnder this couert I shall see, and not be seene" (II.i.45–47).

People who find nothing sinister in playing dress-up tend only to notice the blasphemous implications of Overdo's ambitions, but for a man like Jonson, who seems throughout his career to have regarded the theater with a suspicious eye, these words must surely have carried another set of meanings. Overdo disguises himself not to imitate an other but to "go invisible"—a vital distinction. Those who hide themselves from others' sight deny moral reciprocity with those on whom they are able to spy. In asserting his privilege to see and not be seen, Overdo asserts his right to judge and not be judged. Jonson questions not Overdo's mask as such, nor even his blasphemy, but the motives of someone who "goes invisible" not simply to hide from other men but to judge them—as spectator judges player. Overdo believes, in other words, that he can attend the world as if it were a theatrical performance. In attempting to make the fair into a theater for his eyes only, Overdo takes a moral position as foolish as that of Cokes, who freely immerses himself in the fair's activities.

Here the exclusive poles of festivity and judgment do not fully define the moral nexus of Jonsonian comedy. The result is that *Bartholomew Fair* enacts a basic dilemma of satiric comedy. The element of comic theater that fosters the necessary critical disengagement of viewer from viewed proves to be the source of serious error. The attempt to contemplate folly turns out to be even greater folly. It is as if the very means of knowing were flawed—as if *Bartholomew Fair* formed a graphic demonstration of Bacon's Idols of the Tribe, or (to use a different analogy) a Renaissance equivalent of Heisenberg's "uncertainty principle." The problem that Jonson here investigates is not bad theater or ignorant audiences. The fault lies deeper, in human institutions or in human faculties themselves. Any surveillance discredits any watcher, Jonson seems to be saying, and theater therefore discredits absolutely. For comic theater, where critical detachment from the players is often taken to be a norm, this position is especially significant. Comedy, by converting spectating into an institution, deceives viewers as to the depth of their involvement with the things they see.

Bartholomew Fair addresses this issue at many points by depicting instances in which actors take revenge upon audiences who try to remain beyond reach. No sooner does one fairgoer try to play the role of spectator than a group of participants turn on him and defile him. Overdo stupidly mistakes horsecoursers for cutpurses and cutpurses for civil young men, effectively satirizing his attempt to see and not be seen. The people who assemble to watch Nightingale perform his ballads do not realize that they are themselves being seen by the keen eyes of a hunter who marks them for prey: "And 'i your singing, you must vse your hawks eye nimbly," the thief Edgworth instructs Nightingale, "and flye the purse to a marke, still, where 'tis worne, and o' which side; that you may gi' me the signe with your beake, or hang your head that way i' the tune" (II.iv.42–45).

Even Quarlous and Winwife, Jonson's sometime choral figures, cannot always remain detached from events. Quarlous and Winwife very closely resemble Jonson's actual audience for comedy in that they visit the Fair specifically to observe human folly. "Well," comments Winwife, at the close of the first Act, "I will leaue the chase of my widdow, for to day, and directly to the *Fayre*. These flies cannot, this hot season, but engender vs excellent creeping sport" (I.v.138–41).

Later, arriving at the fair, they behave like spectators who have just entered a playhouse and are waiting for a piece of theater to commence:

> WIN. Wee are heere before 'hem, me thinkes.
> QVAR. All the better, we shall see 'hem come in now.
> [II.v.1–3]

But Leatherhead's raucous cries rudely jolt the complacent esthetes: "What doe you lacke, Gentlemen, what is't you lacke? a fine Horse? a Lyon? a Bull? a Beare? a Dog, or a Cat? an excellent fine *Bartholmew*-bird? or an Instrument? what is't you lacke?" (II.v.4–7). The players' reality not only insists on being heard but also finds a way to assault the would-be spectators and to graft itself onto them; as Quarlous himself informs his companion, "our very being here makes vs fit to be demanded, as well as others" (II.v.17–18). The distinction between spectator and participant which Quarlous and Winwife would maintain cannot long remain unchallenged. Shortly afterward, Quarlous loses his temper during a foolish dispute with Dan Jorden Knockem and clubs his opponent, proving that even the most detached wit cannot play over the fair without becoming deeply implicated in the very things it would mock. Having strolled idly onto the stage intending to play the role of amused spectators, Quarlous and Winwife suddenly discover that they must flee for their lives, pursued by Ursula and her scalding pan.

This recurring encounter between seers and seen enacts something close to combat. Jonson scripts his comedy as a series of spoiled surveillances or monitorings. The *real* comedy develops as a consequence of the failure of the onstage and offstage audiences successfully to frame—to "plot"—their own sequence of events. For Jonson's moral comedy this development has profound implications: the playwright may here be acknowledging that comedy cannot teach spectators by exposing them to folly. We enter the playhouse, as Quarlous and Overdo attend the fair, for fun and profit and above all to judge: and yet our judgment is always befouled by the drunkard's spittle or by the vomit on our shoes. Possibly Jonson's aim with *Bartholomew Fair,* had he wanted to express it discursively, was, as Douglas Duncan suggests, to cause an audience "to resist the boisterous comic spirit with a part of our minds."[18] But Jonson's comedy seems less a conscious indictment of festivity than a grandiloquent and fully open essay on Dionysian madness.

The shifting and manifold images of actors and audiences do not in *Bartholomew Fair* define a static relationship, therefore, nor do they represent Jonson's conception of an ideal. Rather together they create a dynamic which for Jonson and his audience renders both visible and plausible the quintessence of theater. Within this larger scheme, the representative spatial groupings of characters which I have just discussed comprise only a small portion of the comedy. They serve merely to embody, we might say, the "message" of this play, namely, that the fair has no clearly predictable effect on those who attend it except that *any* attempt to use it for specific ends invariably fails. And fail it must, for every onlooker, whether onstage or off: onstage fairgoers cannot remain aloof from the action, and similarly Jonson's Bankside audience is forced to sympathize, to judge, to plot sequences of action, and then is mocked for its folly.

To illustrate this psychology in greater detail we may consider the place of Littlewit's puppet play within the overall design of Jonson's comedy. The playlet and its reception describe a condensed version of *Bartholomew Fair* and its public. Unlike, say, the celebratory playlets which compose the last acts of *Love's Labour's Lost* or *A Midsummer Night's Dream,* this play within the play develops logically from the preceding action. In fact its performance completes one of the five main lines of Jonson's plot. Near the end of Act I (though by Act V not many spectators will remember the lines in question), Littlewit announces to Win his motive in attending the fair: "We must to the *Fayre* too, you, and I, *Win.* I haue an affaire i' the *Fayre, Win,* a Puppet-play of mine owne making, say nothing, that I writ for the *motion* man, which you must see, *Win*" (I.v.145–48). An audience hears nothing more about Littlewit's authorial ambitions until V.iii, when Filcher tries to charge Littlewit money to see his own play. Sharkwell corrects him: "What, doe you not know the *Author,* fellow *Filcher?* you must take no money of him; he must come in *gratis:* Mr. *Littlewit* is a voluntary; he is the *Author*" (20–22).

Like many other apparently random events in the play, this incident demonstrates upon careful inspection the poet's incredible mastery of detail. By reexamining the end of Act I we discover that Jonson clearly and competently "prepared" his audience for this development, and commentators sometimes cite this and scores of similar instances as proof of the artistic unity of *Bartholomew Fair.* "Unity" indeed accurately describes the result of Jonson's meticulous art, but the term is nevertheless highly misleading. Three full acts—nearly two hours' playing time—intervene between Littlewit's description of his play and its actual performance, and the spectator who lacks a copy of the text may surely be forgiven, especially when we consider the extraordinary complexity of the fair's events, if he or she forgets the reason why Littlewit attended the fair in the first place. Jonson does not simply reintroduce Littlewit's play when the audience *least* expects it but also forces the spectators to acknowledge it when they *cannot possibly* expect it. The secret of the "plot" of *Bartholomew Fair* is that an audience experiences it partly as a threat. The induction, the complex intertwinings of characters' motives, the performers' relentless attack on the fairgoers—all represent aspects of an overall assault on an audience. T. S. Eliot once said that *Bartholomew Fair* had "hardly a plot at all,"[19] but as an experiment in histrionic performance the drama indeed possesses a plot, and the onstage fairgoers are not the only spectators who are its victims.

The events of *Bartholomew Fair* are nominally consistent with the logical probability that "unity of plot" requires, and yet they have quite the opposite effect. Kenneth Burke's analysis of *Hamlet* shows how dramatic form may be described in terms of the expectations of the audience, and his discussion of the scene in which Hamlet first confronts his father's ghost provides some terms to clarify the working of the plot of *Bartholomew Fair*.[20] Burke explains that Shakespeare first causes his audience to anticipate seeing the ghost, then deliberately forestalls its entrance on stage, in the meantime subjecting the audience to the noises of an unseen party and Hamlet's lengthy disquisition on the Danish national character. The delay seems at first inexplicable: why would a playwright prepare for a character's imminent entrance (a ghost, no less!) and then not follow through? Burke's explanation of dramatic form in this scene takes into account the emotional needs of the audience. "Form in literature," he writes in one of his memorable definitions, "is an arousing and fulfillment of desires";[21] it is "the creation of an appetite in the mind of the auditor, and the adequate satisfying of that appetite."[22] Thus the form of this particular scene of *Hamlet,* as Burke explains, is superbly correct; in it Shakespeare balances anticipation so exquisitely with disappointment that audiences see the ghost at precisely that moment when they least expect it and yet most yearn for it.

However much we may marvel at Jonson's skill in knitting the raveled ends of his plot, we cannot maintain that Littlewit's play is reintroduced at the moment when an auditor most desires it. In fact spectators are likely to be vexed rather than pleased by its appearance, for its reintroduction touches off within them an unsettling reaction that is difficult to characterize but might be identified by psychologists as a form of paramnesia. *Why now?* they say; *why so long lain dormant?* Dramatic form in *Bartholomew Fair* almost always proves to be the *wrong* form, insofar as the term describes conventional patterns by which an appetite for certain events is aroused and gratified. Jonson reintroduces Littlewit's play not when the spectators most desire it but when they have in fact ceased absolutely to desire it and when its sudden presence reinforces their ignorance. Were this an isolated occurrence we might write it off as an accident, but the sequence involving Littlewit's play actually epitomizes the defiant obscurity of Jonson's plot, as if the playwright were aggressively pursuing a point.

Jonson's point is intentionally disruptive. He interposes digressive material between the initial plotting of a series of events and their affective or intellectual fulfillment in very many sequences. Just before Littlewit's play is announced in Act V, for example, Overdo appears on stage, dressed like a porter, talking like Jehovah, and loudly proclaiming, "Two maine works I haue to prosecute" (V.ii.6–7). But Overdo only elucidates the first of these works before his discourse is interrupted by the entrance of Winwife, Grace, and Quarlous, who is now dressed in the habit of Troubleall. Thus viewers are denied the completion of the sequence which Jonson had caused them to expect. Instead they focus on another of Jonson's plot sequences—the romantic competition between Winwife and Quarlous for the hand of Grace Wellborn. Troubleall (is it not disorienting to be reminded of it at this moment?) had earlier (IV.iii) marked "Palemon," or Winwife's word, on Grace's ballot sheet, but Jonson had withheld this information until now, when, as Grace so aptly puts it, "twere vaine to disguise it longer" (V.ii.30). At this point we are less than thrilled to learn that Winwife is the lucky man, because too much time and action have intervened between the announcement of the contest and the announcement of the winner. In the opening lines of this plot sequence an audience indeed hears the promise of the close, but the playwright gratifies desires for closure only in a way that, in contrast to the psychology of our involvement with respect to the *Hamlet* "ghost" sequence, is strangely perfunctory, meaningless. Going to watch *Bartholomew Fair* is a little like lending money to a forgetful in-law; by the time the investment is recovered, it has been given up for lost. In both cases the contract is technically fulfilled, and yet the experience is not gratifying in the conventional sense. If anything, it is a learning process: we will be a little more wary, in the future, of in-laws and playwrights. This particular scene is twice disorienting, for the episode closes with an ironic twist when Overdo completes the logical circuit that seemed irreparably broken: "Now, for my other worke, reducing the young man (I haue follow'd so long in loue) from the brinke of his bane, to the center of safety" (V.ii.132–34). The lesson for spectators resembles that which Overdo then pronounces, namely, never presume, but learn to "waite the good time" (V.ii.135–36).

Jonson makes the spectator aware of his own commitment to the dramatic performance; this renewed emphasis on the theatrical frame is enacted in miniature by the staging of Littlewit's puppet play. Littlewit's show is rather immodestly titled "the ancient moderne history of *Hero,* and *Leander,* otherwise called *The Touchstone of true Loue,* with as true a tryall of friendship, betweene *Damon* and *Pithias,* two faithfull friends o' the Bankside" (V.iii.6–10). Cokes inquires whether or not the play is an "Enterlude," and the implication, therefore, is that an audience is going to be treated to something like Bottom and company's laughably inept playlet in *A Midsummer Night's Dream.* To restrict the meaning of Littlewit's play in this fashion by classifying it is a discrediting of theater of the same order that tempted onlookers in the induction. The original romantic legend is made to seem merely "playful," the heroic tale of Hero and Leander being metamorphosed "to a more familiar straine for our people" (V.iii.116–17). Littlewit exchanges the Hellespont for the Thames, Leander becomes a dyer's son, and Hero becomes a Bankside wench. Finally, Leatherhead, who is in charge of the performance, reminds Littlewit that plays are things of little account: "I warrant you Sir," he says, "doe not you breed too great an expectation of it, among your friends: that's the onely hurter of these things" (V.iv.12–14).

Any viewers who begin to be lulled by this genial Shakespearean atmosphere are soon awakened. In the first place, there seems to be something gravely wrong with the onstage audience: Whit enters, thoroughly drunk, requesting loudly that "the Mashter o' de *Monshtersh,* helpe a very sicke Lady, here, to a chayre, to shit in" (V.iv.28–29). Nor is the puppets' dialogue especially uplifting, once the play gets under way:

PVP. L.	*Cole, Cole, old Cole.*
LAN.	*That is the Scullers name without controle.*
PVP. L.	*Cole, Cole, I say, Cole.*
LAN.	*We doe heare you.*
PVP. L.	*Old Cole.*
LAN.	*Old cole? Is the Dyer turn'd Collier? how do you sell?*
PVP. L.	*A pox o' your manners, kisse my hole here, and smell.*
LAN.	*Kisse your hole, and smell? there's manners indeed.*
	[V.iv. 128–136]

As Littlewit's play proceeds, Jonson increasingly draws viewers' attention to the effect that the puppets are having on Cokes. In this scene Jonson first offers a graphic account of the effect of players on a naive spectator, one who (Sir Philip Sidney notwithstanding) cannot tell a fictional representation of Thebes, so to speak, from the real one. The playwright dramatizes an eager but ignorant audience; as Cokes earlier defined his position, "I am in loue with the *Actors* already, and I'll be allyed to them presently" (V.iii.131–32).

And so he is. Cokes is at first confused by the performance of the puppets; he needs tutoring in order to understand what is occurring. "What was that, fellow?" he asks Leatherhead, interrupting the play; "Pray thee tell me, I scarce vnderstand 'hem" (V.iv.145–46). But he proves to be a bright student and quickly learns to follow the puppets' dialogue: "He sayes he is no *Pandar*," he interjects at one point: " 'Tis a fine language; I vnderstand it, now" (V.iv.163–64). And he soon responds to the actors with enthusiasm:

PVP. C.	*Harme watch, harme catch.*
COK.	Harme watch, harme catch, he sayes: very good i' faith, the Sculler had like to ha' knock'd you, sirrah.
LAN.	Yes, but that his fare call'd him away.
PVP. L.	*Row apace, row apace, row, row, row, row.*
LAN.	*You are knauishly loaden, Sculler, take heed where you goe.*
PVP. C.	*Knaue i' your face, Goodman Rogue.*
PVP. L.	*Row, row, row, row, row, row.*
COK.	He said knaue i' your face, friend.
LAN.	I sir, I heard him. But there's no talking to these watermen, they will ha' the last word.

COK. God's my life! I am not allied to the Sculler, yet; hee shall be *Dauphin* my boy. But my Fiddle-sticke do's fiddle in and out too much; I pray thee speake to him, on't: tell him, I would haue him tarry in my sight, more.

Especially interesting is Cokes's reaction to staged violence:

COK. How is't friend, ha' they hurt thee?
LAN. O no!
Betweene you and I Sir, we doe but make show.
Thus Gentles you perceiue, without any deniall,
    'twixt Damon *and* Pythias *here, friendships true tryall.*
Though hourely they quarrell thus, and roare each with other,
    they fight you no more, then do's brother with brother.
But friendly together, at the next man they meet,
    they let fly their anger, as here you might see't.
COK. Well, we haue seen't, and thou hast felt it, whatsoeuer thou sayest, what's next? what's next?

[V.iv.277–87]

These exchanges contain several striking points. Cokes, for example, is talking about the process of audience identification, the psychology by which a spectator becomes "allied with" the actor on the stage. Or in the second passage, we might observe the ambiguity of Leatherhead's analogy, "they fight you no more, than do's brother with brother"—surely an allusion to the world's first murderer and first corpse. Also significant is Cokes's ambivalent response to the players' hostilities. Possibly he misunderstands that the violence is fictional and so is troubled by it, yet he overrides whatever misgivings he feels ("thou hast felt it, whatsoeuer thou sayest") and hungers for more ("what's next? what's next?").

Cokes's ignorance of the stage is as profound as his desire for it is keen, and we are therefore tempted to write Cokes off as a representative of the rude spectator whom Jonson constantly labored to instruct. Certainly audiences laugh at Cokes's stupidity, at the sight of this "natural simpleton going through the fair with the spontaneous enthusiasms of a child on a lark."[23] But it is not always easy for spectators to keep their own enlightened responses to the players clearly separate from those of the benighted Cokes.

Festive Comedy: *Bartholomew Fair* 89

Consider, for example, the process of affective responses which the following passage organizes:

> PVP. H. *O* Leander, Leander, *my deare, my deare* Leander,
> *I'le for euer be thy goose, so thou'lt be my gander.*
> COK. Excellently well said, *Fiddle,* shee'll euer be his goose, so hee'll be her gander: was't not so?
> LAN. Yes, Sir, but marke his answer, now.
> PVP. L. *And sweetest of geese, before I goe to bed,*
> *I'll swimme o're the* Thames, *my goose, thee to tread.*
> COK. Braue! he will swimme o're the *Thames,* and tread his goose to[o]night, he sayes.
>
> [V.v.295–304]

During this scene spectators' overall response to the puppets blends very subtly with those of Cokes, partly because he expresses their reaction to Leander's obscene pun on "tread." We might, with Freud, cite this particular joke as an example of tendency wit aimed at sexual exhibition; the pleasure the audience finds in the pun depends on its ability publicly to repeat the forbidden word.

Thus Cokes leads the spectators through the pleasure of the joke. Even though he probably does not himself comprehend the pun, he voices the necessary repetition, completing almost simultaneously the mental circuit which is necessary for the joke to have its full effect on an audience. The implications for Jonson's comic theater are important. In this instance Cokes is clearly not "distanced" from the audience by his folly but in fact acts as an extension of its newly formed communal mind.

Can we deny that Jonson here casts the role of the viewer as inflexibly as that of the performer? And who, in that case, is more foolish? A psychodynamic view of Cokes reveals that fundamental reorientations are taking place with respect to the extent of spectators' involvement in the action. There is enlightened laughter, to be sure, but also rudimentary modes of identification as an audience begins to give itself over to Cokes. This process of identification is intensified once Zeal-of-the-Land Busy begins to dispute with Leatherhead and the voices of the puppets. Busy offers spectators an even greater fool to mock and thus, in terms of the dynamics of their response to the performers, effectively reassigns

Cokes the full measure of the onlookers' desire. Once the intense debate between Busy and the players is under way, the audience becomes witness to a combat and the dynamics of that obvious conflict require the spectators to differentiate their affections very sharply, dividing the actors on stage into "good guys" and "bad guys" whose respective victories and defeats they experience as their own.[24] Jonson here compels his audience to form a group whose various individual psychologies become united in a single common and aggressively hostile will to defeat Busy. In the development of this group madness—not too strong a word—Cokes cannot ever seem to refrain from forming an audience of one and takes on a choric function. He becomes the principal agent in the forming of a highly contagious group mind—a kind of Renaissance cheerleader. Cokes, the fool, here becomes the instrument of spectators' aggressions, and they are "allied" with him:

>Well disputed, Hobby-horse! [V.v.64]
>Good, by my troth, he has giuen him the lye thrice. [V.v.102]
>That's braue i' faith, thou hast carryed it away,
>Hobby-horse, on with the Play! [V.v.118–19]

Thus the staging of the puppet show again manifests the general tendency of Jonson's players to exercise centripetal pull upon an unsuspecting audience. As Cokes becomes lost in the mock combat, so Jonson's Bankside audience yields its judgment to the group mind that the induction so specifically warns against: "It is also agreed, that euery man heere, exercise his owne Iudgement, and not censure by *Contagion,* or vpon *trust,* from anothers voice, or face, that sits by him, be he neuer so first, in the *Commission of Wit*" (97–100). Ironically, at the very moment when spectators are fooled into thinking that the puppets have won the debate and will continue their play, Jonson almost sadistically destroys it. Suddenly Overdo, who has been out of the action for some long period of time, discovers himself and demands an end to all metamorphoses: "Stay, now do I forbid," he roars; "I, *Adam Ouerdoo!* sit still, I charge you" (V.v.120–21).

If the purpose of Jonson's final act is to endorse "festivity," it seems odd that he permits Overdo this unexpected outburst. Spectators have just experienced Busy's defeat as if it were their own triumph. That victory seems complete, as Busy professes to be both chastened and converted to an ardent playgoer: "Let it goe on," he says of the puppets' play; "For I am changed, and will become a beholder with you!" (V.v.116–17). Why should Jonson labor to satirize Puritan zealots, in other words, if he is not going to permit the more enlightened members of his audience to savor the fruits of victory?

At least two answers to this question suggest themselves immediately. The first must be that Jonson himself has a streak of Puritan loathing for the theater and might therefore be reluctant to declare the debate a rout. Alternatively, we might argue with Beaurline that a coup de theatre such as that which Overdo enacts would have delighted Jacobean spectators and that his final tableau could have permitted Jonson's audience "an extra moment of detachment to look back at the drama from an oblique perspective and to reflect upon it, if they were so inclined."[25] Indeed, there is some truth to Beaurline's observation: for the elation felt during these brief moments is intensely, expressly theatrical. It is thrilling to identify with Overdo's desire to see the entire stage arrayed as a panorama; the lure of the spectacle is indeed powerful. "Stay," "Stand forth," "Stand you there," he commands the rest of the company, exactly as if their only reason for being there in front of him were to serve his visual pleasure.

This time, however, spectators do not mock Overdo's folly for attempting to make the world a stage; now they identify with it. In this comic theater, unfortunately, there are no privileged playgoers, neither onstage nor off; and there is considerable risk in sharing Overdo's pleasure at this point. No sooner has he choreographed the scene to his liking than his wife vomits at his feet.

Thus the meaning of this scene accords perfectly with the values that Jonson has pursued throughout the rest of the play. Here, as elsewhere, the poet first tempts his audience to indulge their desire for spectacle. Once more the onlookers surrender unwittingly to the push and pull of a world they believed they could observe merely; and one more time Jonson's plot attacks their ignorance and their moral shortsightedness. The Jacobean stage was capable of intense visual effects, but the moment when Mistress

Overdo vomits at her husband's feet is surely one of the most visually *arresting* moments in all Renaissance theater. Her vomit is the perfect emblem of the celebrants' revenge, proving in a single extravagant gesture that no one can attend to a performance without becoming involved. Beaurline suggests that this emblem reminds Overdo, as he resumes judicial powers, to be "gentle" in his meting out of justice, but the lesson (if that is the word for it) which Jonson here dramatizes has implications far more sweeping.[26] To the extent that we identify with Overdo's yearning for panorama, we again suffer the consequences of secret monitoring. Like much theater, *Bartholomew Fair* is a game, but this game is played against anyone who cannot see that in the theater everyone is a player. *Bartholomew Fair* is the perfect expression of Renaissance drama: it is the comedy par excellence of the theater's deregulation, and audiences are here sullied one last time by one of the players they thought it safe to watch.

The play metaphor in *Bartholomew Fair*, then, is not intended to promote theatrical consciousness, nor to assert festivity and role playing as life-restoring tonics, nor yet to encourage audiences to mend their own lives through the objective contemplation of fools. Rather this drama may be understood as the playwright's effort to relocate comic theater firmly within a moral context. Jonson's approach in this play is exploratory; the play confirms no single answer to the questions it raises, nor—and here it differs from the earlier great Jonsonian comedies—does it provide a single major role that condenses for an audience the central experience of the play. Hence it may be worthwhile to examine *Bartholomew Fair* in order to discover the consequences of eliminating the typical "comic hero."

"Wee'll ha' the rest o' the Play at home"

Of all the many characters in *Bartholomew Fair*, only Quarlous and Winwife manage to achieve anything like the familiar triumphs with which Aristophanes and Plautus often rewarded their protagonists' play. Both are gentlemen wits, both receive brides at the play's end. This familiar package of wit and sex makes Quarlous and Winwife the logical candidates for hero of the comedy. Of the pair, Quarlous is further honored by being granted the privilege of stating Jonson's final piece of advice: "and remember," he tells Overdo, "you are but *Adam,* Flesh, and blood! you haue your frailty, forget your other name of Ouerdoo, and inuite vs all to supper" (V.vi.96–98). In the midst of the tumultuous world of *Bartholomew Fair,* we clutch such bits of apparent rationality as if they were gold, and we are therefore tempted to believe that Quarlous, at least, is meant to have the audience's approval.[27] But before making Quarlous into the poet's raisonneur, we ought to notice that Quarlous slyly seeks more than supper: once at home, he tells Overdo, "There you and I will compare our *discoueries:* and drowne the memory of all enormity in your bigg'st bowle at home" (V.vi.99–100).

Quarlous wants to bring the celebration home, a desire which in itself ought to suggest that there are serious differences between his opinions and those of Jonson. A more important objection to Quarlous's candidacy for raisonneur status, however, is the fact that it proves impossible neatly to divide *Bartholomew Fair* into characters with whom onlookers "identify" and fools whom they consistently scorn. Indeed the comedy works partly by confusing familiar patterns of empathy and judgment which must have been familiar to Jonson's audience for comedy. Lacking a strong centralizing persona with which they can consistently align their own interests or criticisms, Jonson's spectators regularly change the locus of their psychic investment. This process involves them in considerable risks and requires them frequently to play the role of onlooker, which in this comedy invariably turns out to be the fool's role. That Quarlous and Winwife are in the long run less foolish than Overdo and Cokes does not of itself establish that Jonson intended his audience to sympathize with the former pair and withhold sympathy from the latter. In fact, as the language of the puppet play suggests, the slippery nature of an audience's sympathies itself seems to be the primary object of the poet's concern.

Some participatory psychology seems critical to spectators' experience of drama, but it is not at all clear on which side of the footlights the motive for this process originates. It is by no means clear, for example, that spectators identify with certain characters only because the playwright has built clear moral differences into his drama. Many people believe that dramatists intentionally control the "sympathies" of the audience by deploying the "good" characters against the "bad" ones, but a drama like *Bartholomew Fair* (and certainly any sports event) suggests rather that the necessary differentiating identifications originate partly in the minds of the beholders. Audiences, being audiences, will identify with (or will "sympathize with," to use that less accurate term) wise men just as readily as with fools—which seems to be Jonson's point.

Exactly why audiences cannot remain apart from actors is a subject beyond the scope of this book. I mention it only to highlight crucial differences between the many actor/characters with whom spectators identify in *Bartholomew Fair* and those whose moral perspective Jonson means an audience to share, which are nonexistent. Spectators are indeed likely to find Quarlous's motives more reasonable than, say, those of Cokes or Overdo. But it does not follow that Quarlous provides spectators with an ideal critical perspective on the play's events. The script compels spectators repeatedly to merge their interests with any character who happens at that moment to be dominating the stage by playing audience to the action. For these reasons, *Bartholomew Fair* might profitably be read as an experiment in the psychology of the audience. As *Volpone,* in Thomas Greene's excellent summation, is "an anatomy of metamorphosis,"[28] so *Bartholomew Fair* is an anatomy of theater psychology, a brilliant disquisition on the theater event and its meaning as a social institution.

That Jonson focuses his comedy upon a Dionysian psychology does not mean that he wholeheartedly endorses it. For this reason, possibly, he gives the last words of the play to Cokes, surely the character who is most foolish in his worship of the players: "Yes, and bring the *Actors* along, wee'll ha' the rest o' the *Play* at home" (V.vi.114–15). It is brilliantly ironic that Jonson permits Cokes to utter the benediction on *Bartholomew Fair,* and surely we do not dare equate his foolish enthusiasm with Jonson's own position. Cokes cannot possibly profit from the theater because he commits himself wholeheartedly to the actors' fiction. As Waspe scolds him during one of the puppets' brawls, "They lack'd but you to be their second, all this while" (V.iv.357–58). Yet before concluding that any other character offers a more reliable position, we should examine the epilogue which Jonson wrote for the play's second performance. Jonson does not specify who speaks the epilogue, which is addressed specifically to James I:

> *Your* Maiesty *hath seene the* Play, *and you*
> *can best allow it from your eare, and view.*
> *You know the scope of* Writers, *and what store*
> *of* leaue *is giuen them, if they take not more,*
> *And turne it into* licence: *you can tell*
> *if we have vs'd that* leaue *you gaue vs, well:*
> *Or whether wee to* rage, *or* license *breake,*
> *or be* prophane, *or make* prophane *men speake?*
> *This is your power to iudge (great Sir) and not*
> *the enuy of a few. Which if wee haue got,*
> *Wee value lesse what their dislike can bring,*
> *if it so happy be, t' haue pleas'd the* King.

Jonson's motives in adding the epilogue to his comedy can only be guessed at. Possibly he thought that by flattering James he might forestall charges that his play satirized the monarch: after all, James's disliking for pork was widely known, as was his opposition to tobacco (the king had in 1604 published *A Counterblaste to Tobacco*). The possibility was indeed real, therefore, that James might read malice in Busy's frantic campaign against pigs and Overdo's condemnation of tobacco.

It is significant, nevertheless, that the ending to *Bartholomew Fair* differs markedly from other instances of Jonsonian dramatic closure. Consider the ending of *Volpone:*

> The seasoning of a play is the applause.
> Now, though the FOX be punish'd by the lawes,
> He, yet, doth hope, there is no suffring due,
> For any fact, which he hath done 'gainst you;

> If there be, censure him: here he, doubtfull, stands.
> If not, fare iovially, and clap your hands.
>
> [*Works* 5:136]

Or of *Epicoene:*

> Spectators, if you like this *comoedie,* rise
> cheerefully, and now MOROSE is gone in, clap your hands.
> It may be, that noyse will cure him, at least please him.
>
> [*Works* 5:271]

Or of *Every Man in his Humor* or *The Alchemist:*

> BRAYNE-WORME! to whom all my addresses
> of courtship shall haue their reference. Whose aduentures,
> this day, when our grand-children shall heare to be made a
> fable, I doubt not, but it shall find both spectators, and
> applause.
>
> [*Works* 3:402]

>   Gentlemen,
> My part a little fell in this last *Scene,*
> Yet 'twas *decorum.* And though I am cleane
> Got off from SVBTLE, SVRLY, MAMMON, DOL,
> Hot ANANIAS, DAPPER, DRVGGER, all
> With whom I traded; yet I put my selfe
> On you, that are my countrey: and this pelfe
> Which I haue got, if you doe quit me, rests
> To feast you often, and inuite new ghests.
>
> [*Works* 5:407]

In each of these instances Jonson clearly aligns his audience with respect to the protagonist and to his play. To arraign the actor in this fashion before the audience is to acknowledge the terms of the theater's contract, to complete the gestures by which the fictions of the playhouse are framed with respect to the realities of the departing audience. The aim is to bring the spectators and players critically to bear on each other, and Jonson's audience must surely have come to expect such explicit recognitions to bracket the theater with respect to the rest of society.

But what of the ending to *Bartholomew Fair?* The entire comedy has been building to this moment of apparent celebration; every last fairgoer has become a celebrant. The final triumphant

Festive Comedy: *Bartholomew Fair*   97

exodus looses the mass of players into England's streets and houses. For once, Jonson seems to endorse the players and the theater, and yet the terms of that endorsement are ambiguous. The stage is empty. Spectators are silent. Jonson does not bracket the play by writing viewers' applause into the ending of his comedy. For that matter, he does not acknowledge the presence of an audience, addressing, at some unspecified point after the last actor has left the stage, only King James.

However much time must elapse between the actors' exodus and the speaking of the epilogue (who comes forward to speak these lines? the poet himself?, Jonson surely cannot have intended his spectators immediately to explode the playhouse with noise. Indeed the effect is quite unlike the typical end of Renaissance comic theater. The swiftly emptied stage, the lack of an actor who formally closes the drama by acknowledging the audience and begging their applause, the dwindling offstage cheerings which deepen the spectators' awareness of their own isolated silence—all these elements of the performance leave spectators with an uncanny awareness that it is time to play *their* role. But now, suddenly, they are also aware that there is no script to guide them. And Jonson insists that his audience experience this self-consciousness; he wants them one last time to feel the theatrical frame beginning to come unstuck, so to speak, before he lets them leave the playhouse.

It is a disquieting experience, an eerie silence unexpectedly sprung upon an audience at the tumultuous conclusion of Jonson's most boisterous comedy. But above all it is an intensely *exhausting* experience, a reminder to the spectators that they must remain chained in their seats until freed by the play. It compels them to acknowledge their role and to understand that their parts have been scripted as surely as those of the actors. The silence forces them ultimately to acknowledge the extent of their involvement with the players. For a brief period (how long between the exodus and the epilogue? ten seconds? fifteen? A silence even longer probably can be justified in the performance), a void opens beneath Jonson's theater, and we sense the mysterious forces which shape the playwright's most daring comedy. Amid the fading noises of the actors' revelry Cokes's last words continue to reverberate in spectators' ears—"wee'll ha' the rest of the *Play* at home." And the accumulated meaning of the entire performance of *Bartholomew Fair* is distilled within that single enigmatic promise, a promise which epitomizes the enigmatic pull of the theater for Jonson as well as for his age.

Thus it is supremely appropriate that an unnamed actor on an empty stage speak an epilogue addressed only to James. The end of *Bartholomew Fair* offers England's king the opportunity earlier extended to spectators and to the surrogate audience on stage. James is now asked to judge the play, "to allow it from . . . eare, and view." It is of course fitting that Jonson locates the theatrical performance specifically in relation to the king, establishing, as it were, the boundaries between theater and society. But from another perspective this ultimate figuration appears just as unstable as all the earlier joinings of actors and audiences.The king functions at this final moment as have all the earlier surrogate audiences. Even though he does not appear on stage, he becomes one more character with a role he must play out. As Cokes, Overdo, Littlewit, and Quarlous in their own individual ways represent attempts to frame a meaningful relationship with the fair, so here the king's presence completes an ultimate gestural figuration of players and spectators.

Certainly, as head of state, the king completes visually the respective orientations of "society" and "festivity," but in this case it is necessary to update the customary interpretation of festive comedy as enacting the mythos of rule and misrule. *Bartholomew Fair* does not clearly demarcate the relative boundaries of pleasure and sobriety, just as James's presence does not symbolically constrain festivity. If the close of *Bartholomew Fair* is intensely aural, it is intensely visual, too. Of course there is no final tableau, no arrangement of actors or lovers or bodies on stage, but that is precisely the point. In the final moments of the play Jonson returns his performance to its beginnings. Once more the audience contemplates an empty stage. And this organizing symbolic perspective—a silent, contemplative gaze—Jonson will have his spectators experience before he permits them to applaud and depart. He publishes the limits of the theatrical frame by denying its conceptual validity.

Experiencing this sensation is a very different thing—and a vastly more important one for Jonson's audience—from learning that there is a time for revelry and a time for sobriety, or that misrule consolidates rule, or even that we must constantly discriminate morally as we view the world's events. *Bartholomew Fair* does not finally resolve the conflict between actors and audiences which it dramatizes. Instead it exemplifies the contradictions inherent in a society that did not fully know how to interpret its own potential for histrionic expression.[29] There is ample evidence in *Bartholomew Fair* to prove that this play is not about festivity but about theater, hence it matters little whether we vote in the end to censure the fairgoers or to join them. Rather an ontological point emerges: for in this comedy Jonson enacts the risks humans incur when they make the world into a stage. The comedy neither embraces the players nor asks spectators to condemn their folly but requires them to grasp a truth more difficult and more equivocal. Nine years earlier Jonson in *Volpone* had taught his audience (as Greenblatt puts it) that they could not remain in the playhouse forever,[30] but *Bartholomew Fair* comes to a more radical conclusion: as the poet discovered in writing *this* comedy, you are a great fool if you think you can attend a play and remain seated safely in the audience.

4 Shamming Illness and Shamming Identity: Doctors and Actors in *Le malade imaginaire*

> Here lies one who is said to be dead. I don't know if he is, or if he is sleeping. His *Malade Imaginaire* could not have caused his death. It is a trick he is playing for fun, because he was fond of shamming. Be that as it may, here lies Molière; since he was a great comedian, if he is acting an imaginary corpse, he does it well.
>
> —one of many contemporary epitaphs commemorating Molière's death

Le malade imaginaire is always remembered with pain because of the macabre paradox of the playwright who turned his own dying into a piece of comic theater. The play is less familiar than the masterpieces of the 1660s—*Tartuffe, L'avare, Le misanthrope*—and modern readers may be bored with all the scatological joking even if they realize that for Molière's audience purges and enemas were not what we might normally term laughing matters. Nevertheless, the play is an excellent choice for a discussion of representative comic theaters because of its explicit concern with attempts to cure the humorous individual. In formal outline, the play follows very closely the pattern normally associated with New Comedy. Such comedy is said normally to be corrective and broadly social: its plot dramatizes an attempt to adjust the behavior of antisocial characters to conform to a known and clearly desirable societal norm. The story of such plays is exceedingly familiar; as Frye once remarked, the plot of New Comedy is "less a form than a formula."[1] If such plays vary little from one another, their audiences are thought to vary even less. According to the standard view, Molière's spectators behave exactly like those of Terence or Menander. They do not expect comic theater to address difficult or profound truths. They come, instead, to reject villainy, laugh at folly, and applaud enthusiastically the social reconciliation which takes place on stage during the closing moments of the play.

Is Molière's play socializing in this way? Does the meaning of this comedy differ in no fundamental way from that typical of its Latin and Greek antecedents? Or do important contradictions between mythos and gestus perhaps distinguish *Le malade imaginaire* from earlier forms of New Comedy? Certainly *Le malade imaginaire* nominally obeys the familiar conventions of the New Comedy formula. But the apparently serene facade masks a problematic and newly flexible exchange of the real and the illusory. The protagonist and his performance gain a dimension, making it more accurate to speak here of a spectrum of representation than of representation itself. J. D. Hubert calls attention to some of the most obvious doublings, all of which would be highly visible to the comedy's seventeenth-century spectators and which are crucial to the experience of it in the theater. They are meant to be seen, and, writes Hubert, they often put spectators in a "piquant situation, partly pleasurable and partly disturbing. Argan is both Molière and not Molière; both a malingerer and a sick man; both a madman who enjoys his imaginary illness and a sufferer who, with barely enough strength to support his disease, has done his utmost to entertain the audience."[2]

Le malade imaginaire vacillates between reality and illusion whether Molière plays Argan or not. The part confronts any actor with a series of interpretive problems designed to stress the impossibility of ever fully integrating the role and the "real" self. My discussion will examine whether such comedy can be classified simply as a "socializing" experience, and the related but more general question of the relationship between theater and therapy. I shall explore a hypothesis by means of which Molière's comedy may be understood as part of a larger and specifically modern (that is, post-Renaissance) discourse on selfhood and mental health.

When the play opens, Argan, the hypochondriac, is seen seated in his bedroom; alone, he methodically reviews his recent payments to doctors and apothecaries. He counts mechanically, talking for a long time to no one but himself:

> Three and two is five, and five is ten, and ten is twenty. Three and two is five. "Plus, on the twenty-fourth, a little enema, insinuating, preparatory, and emollient, to mollify, humidify, and refresh the bowels of the gentleman. . . . Plus, on the same day, a good detergent enema, composed with double catholicon, rhubarb, rose honey, and so on, according to the prescription, to cleanse, bathe, and scour the lower intestine of the gentleman, thirty sous."[3]

Argan's isolation from society is already total. When he talks, no one listens; when he shouts, no one comes; and when he rings for attention, no one hears. Furiously he yells for Toinette, his maidservant, but when she appears onstage, no meaningful communication takes place. Instead, Toinette interrupts her master's every attempt to speak by moaning over a feigned injury. Her maneuver is funny but quite significant. It is the first of many instances in the comedy when hypocrisy is used as a mode of defense or self-aggrandizement:

> ARGAN: Ah, you bitch! you slut . . . !
> TOINETTE, *acting as if she has bumped her head:* Damn your impatience! You hurry people so much that I got a big blow on the head against the edge of the shutter.
> ARGAN, *angered:* Ah! you villain . . . !
> TOINETTE, *always interrupting and hindering his shouts by groaning:* Ah!
> ARGAN: It is. . . .
> TOINETTE: Ah!
> ARGAN: It is an hour. . . .
> TOINETTE: Ah!
> ARGAN: You left me. . . .
> TOINETTE: Ah!

[Pp. 1101–2]

Two things are satirized in this introductory sequence of scenes. Argan is first imaged in the context of disease, as he recites a veritable inventory of contemporary methods for dealing with illness. The picture Molière draws of medical practice is not greatly exaggerated. Disease was thought in the seventeenth century to be essentially a problem of cleansing, and the average physician therefore pursued a course of evacuative treatments for nearly every kind of malady. Bleeding, purging, enemas—all were commonly prescribed to rid the body of various noxious humors. Argan's dependency on his physicians is rendered as satire on contemporary reality: whatever they may have thought of their own personal physicians, the audience would have found Argan's behavior laughable.

Next to the farcical attack on the medical profession, however, lies a more important satiric target—Argan. Certainly he behaves like a fool because of his hypochondria. But an even graver folly is his absolute isolation from society. Indeed he cannot even participate in the most elemental dialogue; his sentences are cut short, rendered utterly ineffective by Toinette's feigned moans. Taking the first two scenes of the comedy in concert, we could hardly ask for a more graphic rendering of asocial conduct. Clearly Argan is consumed by a range of "sicknesses" which somebody must undertake to cure.

When communication between Argan and Toinette at last proceeds, there develops a complication familiar to audiences of New Comedy. Older and younger generations disagree as to who should marry whom: Angélique, Argan's elder daughter, loves a young man (Cléante), who plans to ask for her hand. But their marriage is blocked by Argan, who, for obvious practical reasons, has decided to marry his daughter to a physician. Argan's wishes are opposed vigorously by Toinette, and by his second wife, Béline, who hopes to place both of her husband's daughters (by his first wife) in a convent and so to secure any inheritance for herself.

From this point, events swiftly become complex. In Act II, Cléante arrives at Argan's house, disguised as a music teacher, and soon after him come the doctors Diafoirus—father and son Thomas, Angélique's officially approved suitor. Both Cléante and Thomas request Angélique's hand. The action at this point involves a provocative inversion of being and seeming: Cléante and Angélique "play" a pastoral love scene for Argan and his guests. Their playing enables them publicly to avow their love for each other while hiding the truth from Argan, who does not suspect that they mean what they say. Angélique subsequently disavows her father's plans for her marriage. At the end of the second act, as after the first, the story is suspended for the performance of a pastoral ballet. When the action resumes, Toinette and Béralde, Argan's brother, plot to get Angélique the husband she desires. Again the comedy turns to images of play: Toinette masquerades as a doctor and persuades Argan to feign death in order to discover the depths of his family's love. Béline's villainous scheming is thus brought to light, as is Angélique's devotion to her father, and Argan finally agrees to have Cléante as a son-in-law if he will become a doctor. Cléante tentatively agrees, but this requirement is waived when Argan himself is persuaded to become a physician. During a final ballet, several actors, whom Béralde conveniently provides for the occasion, incorporate most of the cast into an impromptu burlesque of the ceremony used to confer a doctor's degree. Argan, now ostensibly cured of his humorous self-centeredness, participates in the communal dancing and singing. As the play ends, everyone onstage seems to join together in the conventional dance of comedy which signifies the inauguration of the new social order.

This is a simplified structural reading of *Le malade imaginaire*. Such an interpretation presupposes that Molière's comedy is accessible on two levels, which narrative theorists might call the separate planes of "content" and "expression."[4] According to this view, there is in every single work of New Comedy a basic "story" which is unchanging and perfectly transportable over time and even across literary modes. Less a skeleton than a scaffold, it constitutes a Platonic abstraction which is independent of any particular New Comedy, even though it governs the hypothetical meaning of all works within the tradition. When all historical and psychological variables have been discarded, so to speak, there still remains of *Le malade imaginaire* a comic "deep structure," a made-in-Greece plot which informs audiences that the forces of darkness and dissolution have been routed by springtime and love and light. From this perspective, *Le malade imaginaire* is said to enact the essential comic mythos by which old societies yield to new ones. This social imperative stands in relation to comedy as a basement to a fully built house; literally, it constitutes an ahistoric and transposable story which is realized (or "actualized" or "expressed") by means of Molière's individual retelling.

Neither the shape nor the source of Molière's plot is in dispute. It can be found little changed in countless older plays, as well as in many newer ones. But hearing a plot summary of a play is not the same experience as seeing the play performed, and we must ask whether or not the meaning of *Le malade imaginaire* is seriously altered by such narrative abstractings.[5] The question is not idle. The closer we approach the protagonists of ancient comedy, for example, the less they seem to be simplistic parodies of the existing order, on the one hand, or univocal celebrants of sex and springtime on the other. Similarly, there exist moments in *Le malade imaginaire* when Argan is neither a comic butt nor a foolish blocking character. There are "watershed moments" in the comedy when he epitomizes a complex realm of attitudes toward theater and problems of individual identity. Actually, the role of Argan is a remarkable and highly sensitive instrument for unlocking a mass of contradictions inherent in the notions of actor and mask, individual and social institution, truth to self and hypocrisy.

Perhaps the first observation to be made regarding *Le malade imaginaire* with respect to earlier versions of New Comedy is that this drama appears to place increased emphasis on hypocritical existence as a social norm. To be sure, in seventeenth-century France acting was considered a disreputable profession— only in 1641 did Louis absolve actors from the charge of infamy inherited from Roman law.[6] But in Plautine comedy, the locus of histrionic force is a hero (the slave) who, because of his powers of self-transformation, clearly dominates the rest of the cast. In *Le malade imaginaire,* on the other hand, it is the de facto hero who is ignorant of plays and pretense.[7] Toinette, Béralde, Cléante, Angélique, and Béline all know how to improvise a script to attain their ends; even little Louison at one point feigns death in order to avoid being beaten by her father. Thus Molière's protagonist strives ironically to learn a truth that everybody else already knows: that in order to be successful one must be able to *play*. In one sense, therefore, this is the subject of *Le malade imaginaire*. Argan moves from fear and isolation in the beginning of the comedy to final immersion in a theatrical event. He cures both hypochondria and misanthropy by reorienting his perspectives to coincide with the majority view: theater, in short, becomes therapy.

For all that, however, the comedy scarcely celebrates theater and its effects; if anything, Molière's attitude toward it is equivocal. Consider one crucial scene of "play within the play," that involving Argan and his younger daughter, Louison; Argan has just learned that Louison has seen her elder sister together with a young man, and he questions her as to her sister's conduct:

> ARGAN: Did I not ask you to come to me first thing to report anything you see?
> LOUISON: Yes, Papa.
> ARGAN: Did you do that?
> LOUISON: Yes, Papa. I came and told you everything I saw.
> ARGAN: And you saw nothing today?
> LOUISON: No, Papa.
> ARGAN: No?
> LOUISON: No, Papa.
> ARGAN: For sure?
> LOUISON: For sure.
> ARGAN: Well then! I'll make you see something.
> *He seizes a switch.*
> LOUISON: Oh! Papa.
> ARGAN: Oh, oh! you little deceiver, you did not tell me that you saw a man in your sister's room.
> LOUISON: Papa!
> ARGAN: I'll teach you to lie.
> LOUISON, *falling on her knees:* Oh! Papa, forgive me. You see, my sister told me not to tell you; but I will tell you everything.
> ARGAN: First you must be whipped on account of lying. Then after that we'll see about the rest.
> LOUISON: Forgive me, Papa!
> ARGAN: No, no.
> LOUISON: Dear Papa, don't whip me!

ARGAN: Now you're going to get it.
LOUISON: In God's name! Papa, don't do it.
ARGAN, *taking her for a whipping:* Come on, come on.
LOUISON: Oh! Papa, you've injured me. Stop: I'm dead. (*She pretends to be dead.*)
ARGAN: Wait! What's this? Louison, Louison. Oh, my God. Louison. Oh! my daughter! Oh! woe, my poor daughter is dead. What have I done, wretch! Oh! Damned whip. Plague take the whip! Oh! my dear daughter, my poor little Louison.
LOUISON: There, there, Papa, don't cry so much, I am not dead quite yet.

[Pp. 1144–45]

Of course this is a funny scene. Moreover, Louison's hypocrisy differs from that of the malicious Béline. It threatens no one; it is spontaneous and harmless—child's play, as opposed to an adult's conniving. Yet Louison's play has its problems. In the first place, the scene adds nothing to the romance of Angélique and Cléante. Next, it introduces an unnecessary character, Louison, who appears nowhere else in the comedy. Finally, there is the question of casting: the role of Louison was created for Louise Beauval, the young daughter of the actors who played Toinette and Thomas Diafoirus.[8] A superfluous scene involving an unnecessary character played by an eight-year-old girl: there is nothing like it in the rest of Molière's oeuvre. Why, therefore, does Molière include it?

As James F. Gaines notes, the scene underscores Argan's social dysfunction (once again he cannot tell truth from illusion) and also "serves to prefigure Toinette's ingenious solution to the problem of medical parasitism."[9] But the scene yields additional, fascinating resonances. The episode is structured so that Argan confronts both a small child and (in the 1673 production) a nonprofessional actor. Unless we suppose that Molière risked wasting the scene just to indulge one of the many Beauval children, the playwright's strategy here seems to be twofold. He first introduces a character so young that her innocence is beyond suspicion and requires the role to be played by a person with limited histrionic technique.

It is intriguing, therefore, to consider the ways in which the use of an untrained actor might have been to Molière's advantage.

Why, for example, does "Louison"—the character—decide to "play dead"? To avoid being whipped by her father, we might say. It is a clever ploy: the ultimate form of disqualifying oneself as an *actor* (that is, a participant) is to pretend to be incapable of any action whatsoever. Thus Louison (the fiction), to avoid the physical pain and the psychic stress of being beaten by one she loves, shams death. Of course her action is "childish." But does Louison (the fiction) really fear that she is dying? Perhaps—but suppose that this is not the first time she has been punished by Argan, that this is to her a familiar situation. Might her action not then constitute a sophisticated behavioral mechanism whereby an aggressor is made to cease his attack because his victim has disqualified herself from any further participation in this particular script? Louison's final comment—"I am not quite dead yet"—suggests that she has been pretending all along. And what about the onlookers? Do they not see almost instantly that Louison is shamming? Molière does not want to stage a credible illusion of fear. Rather, the amateur's relatively unsophisticated performance—because it doubtless lacks technique and is therefore "unrealistic"—helps to engage spectators with the actor/character in a knowing deception. The performance invites an audience to see that not simply a child's behavior but an *imitation* of childish behavior is being displayed, the explicit aim of which is to deceive an adult. Louison's recovery does not really surprise an audience; from the spectators' point of view, her resurrection is not a miracle on the order, say, of Hermione's return from the dead at the end of *The Winter's Tale.* Molière's scene emphasizes not only Argan's ignorance but also the sheer spontaneity of Louison's shamming: insofar as she instinctively plays dead, she enacts an exploitative fabrication similar to Toinette's feigned injury or Cléante's pretense to love. It is a strange and revealing moment, all the more so because it is so clearly innocent of conventional theatrical artifice, and for a moment we glimpse the extent of the world's theatricality. From the wicked Béline to the innocent Louison, there is visible a grand spectrum of hypocrisy.

There is, then, among all the characters in *Le malade imaginaire* an essential unity of response to Argan. Only the protagonist seems to act without guile or self-consciousness; nearly everyone else produces hypocritical behavior as the situation demands it. The implication is that an individual may somehow disqualify himself or herself as a full participant in events (sham injury, play dead, act a fiction) in order to achieve an end otherwise unattainable—inheritance, love, freedom from personal injury. Such gestural moments abound in Molière's comedy. But as was true in the case of Louison's feigning, they are rarely integrated with the comic Oedipus plot. More often (as in the case of Toinette's injury or Louison's playing possum) they are gratuitous additions designed to poke fun at Argan because of his fundamental incapacity. Argan is funny because he alone cannot recognize a script, let alone improvise one. Are audiences to understand, therefore, that it is "normal" or "natural" to be able to construct multiple versions of the self?

The question is a source of anxiety on many counts. If the central aim of the comedy is to restore the humorous individual to health, how do we imagine Argan is to be "cured" of his various incapacities? In the case of his hypochondria, it is easy to say what is wrong with him. He must be taught that his illness is not real. When it comes to his inability to "play," however, what error is he supposed to be making? On the basis of the examples of Louison and Toinette, we might say that Argan needs to learn to "pretend" in order to be able to protect himself. But the implications of that statement may not be perfectly satisfactory: is the ability to survive in the world to be gained, then, only by a process of willed creation of imaginary identities? Toinette and Louison and the rest of the characters in the comedy "conduct" or "orchestrate" their identities; are they therefore more "healthy" than Argan, who is merely being?

Images of play and medicine thus fuse to turn *Le malade imaginaire* into an elaborate disquisition on psychobiological methods by which to treat the suffering individual. As both the doctors and the "actors" attempt to effect Argan's return to wholeness and health, their various suggestions and vocabularies are allowed to comment one upon the other, so that some treatments are held out as appropriate and others as ineffective or deleterious. Medicine—medicine as practiced in the fashion of contemporary physicians—not only fails to relieve individual suffering but also exacerbates it.

Against the selfish and destructive efforts of the doctors, Molière sets the play of the actor-physicians, chiefly Toinette and Béralde. Béralde at one point notes the essential similarity of doctors and actors when he tells his brother that theater, in effect, is "good medicine": "As for myself, brother, I don't take on the job of combatting medicine; and everyone, at his own risk and fortune, may believe whatever he pleases. What I'm saying is between us only, and I wish I had been able to enlighten you a little as to your mistakes, and, for your entertainment, to take you to see some of Molière's comedies on this subject" (p. 1155).

At first, as Béralde's advice implies, theater seems effective treatment. Yet when, midway through the comedy, Argan wins his liberation from the doctors, he passes immediately into the hands of an equally rapacious order, that of the actors. Argan eventually discovers that physicians cannot cure him, but in the course of doing so he gives himself up to other "physicians" whose successes are in some ways more profoundly unsettling than the failures of their predecessors. Indeed the theatrical "cure" prescribed for Argan is every bit as murderous as the purges sought by the doctors. What Argan experiences during the course of the comedy is not so much a progressive cure as a substitution. Against the folly of the doctors stands the egocentrism of the actors.

The ruthlessness implicit in this particular play ethic proves disconcerting; ultimately, *Le malade imaginaire* reaches the melancholy conclusion that both medicine and theater are supportive treatments only. Neither relieves individual suffering or the burdens of self-consciousness. In the terms proposed by this comedy, doctors and actors are interchangeable. Both perform violent operations on the individual, and the catharsis which the latter group offers the patient is not that induced by fresh cassia and Levantine senna but rather that purging of noxious portions of self which the theatrical experience is traditionally said to accomplish. Theater is medicine turned inside out, and as regards Argan, both methods are more consumptive than curative. It is hard not to read in the comedy symptoms of a fundamental psychosocial reality. It is as if catharsis is in the very order of things.

Of course Molière elsewhere makes use of these and related

materials,[10] but nowhere in the rest of the canon is the focus so intense. Nowhere else are such deeply theatrical questions realized so stunningly in metaphor. When, for example, Béralde first encounters his brother, he brings him a piece of theater, hoping by it to cure Argan of his malaise. Béralde says: "I'm bringing you an entertainment I found, which will dispel your gloom and put you in a better frame of mind for the things we have to discuss. They are gypsies dressed as Moors, who perform dances mingled with songs, which I am sure will delight you; and they will do more good than one of the prescriptions of Monsieur Purgon. Come on" (p. 1147).

Initially, Argan is rendered laughable by his absolute reliance on the arbitrary and artificial products of human invention. He believes completely in the nonsensical theories of the physicians, and Béralde's solution to his brother's discomfort seems both simple and sound. Argan is to do nothing but let "nature" take its course. "You need do nothing more than rest," he tells Argan. "Nature, by herself, when we let her be, will slowly draw out of the disorder into which she has fallen. It is our own disquiet, our own impatience which spoils everything, and nearly all men die of their cures, and not of their sicknesses" (p. 1154). Argan, Béralde suggests, should rid himself of the absurd coercions of the doctors and trust his well-being to his own spontaneous impulses. Béralde's advice sounds well intentioned, and—when compared to Monsieur Purgon's quackery—has the ring of truth. It is folly to live as Argan does. According to Béralde, "nature" includes within itself an implacable necessity that will restore complete health if only the sufferer submits. "You must bear in mind," he says, "that the principles of your life are in you yourself, and that the wrath of Monsieur Purgon is as little capable of making you die as are his remedies of making you live" (p. 1160).

These are vigorous and persuasive words, yet we cannot accept them at face value. Their worth is negated by the fact that in the very act of uttering them Béralde takes on the role of a physician attempting to cure his patient, despite his own earlier warning to his brother: "Between us, I think it one of the greatest follies among men, and looking at matters as a philosopher. I see nothing more ridiculous than one man who tries to have a hand in curing another" (p. 1152).

Béralde is not the only person who believes that theater is therapy; Toinette also prescribes for the patient a dose of histrionics: "It is necessary to prevent this foolish marriage he has taken into his fancies, and I thought to myself it would be a good idea to be able to bring here a doctor of our own, to disgust him with his Monsieur Purgon, and to discredit his methods. But since we have no one in hand for that purpose, I am resolved to play a trick out of my head" (p. 1150).

Between Toinette and Béralde, and Monsieur Purgon, in fact, there exists considerable professional jealousy. Béralde, concluding a lengthy argument against the efficacy of doctors' cures, asserts that the "facts" of medicine are as ephemeral as the theater's fictions. Doctors beguile patients with "the fiction of medicine" (p. 1154), he tells Argan. "But when you come to truth and experience, you get nothing out of all that, and it is like those lovely dreams which leave you nothing upon waking but grief for having believed them" (p. 1154). As the play develops, the actor/doctor metaphor becomes more and more visible, until finally, in the closing burlesque, it becomes, of course, no longer metaphor but an identity.

In this respect, *Le malade imaginaire* is less a celebration of love than a medical symposium. The subject of debate concerns the relative efficacy of physical and psychical therapists; it is a contest between quacks who want to purge Argan's bowels and mountebanks who want to purge his identity. Both sides meet in the metaphor of the theater. Both sides are alike in the violence which they commit upon their patient in the name of therapy, and the formal signs of the competition are the dramatized rituals in Act III, which mark Argan's transfer from one set of therapists to another. Before the care of Argan's self can be assumed by Béralde and company, the patient, in a scene which clearly parallels the Church's rite of excommunication, is first abandoned by the physicians:

> MONSIEUR PURGON: I must tell you that I abandon you to your bad constitution, to the intemperance of your

bowels, to the corruption of your blood, to the bitterness
of your bile and the feculence of your humors.
TOINETTE: Well done!
ARGAN: My God!
MONSIEUR PURGON: And I swear that within four days you
will reach an incurable state.
ARGAN: Oh! mercy!
MONSIEUR PURGON: That you will fall into bradypepsia . . .
ARGAN: Monsieur Purgon!
MONSIEUR PURGON: From bradypepsia to dyspepsia . . .
ARGAN: Monsieur Purgon!
MONSIEUR PURGON: From dyspepsia to apepsia . . .
ARGAN: Monsieur Purgon!
MONSIEUR PURGON: From apepsia to lientery . . .
ARGAN: Monsieur Purgon!
MONSIEUR PURGON: From lientery to dysentery . . .
ARGAN: Monsieur Purgon!
MONSIEUR PURGON: From dysentery to dropsy . . .
ARGAN: Monsieur Purgon!
MONSIEUR PURGON: And from dropsy to loss of life, to
which your folly will have led you.
ARGAN: Oh, my God! I am dead. My brother, you have done
me in.

[P.1158–59][11]

We cannot be absolutely certain of Molière's intentions, so thoroughly does the scene mingle the various institutions—Church, medicine, theater—created to ensure the psychomatic health of the individual. Whether the source of the conflict here dramatized was finally Molière's own psyche or the tensions of the neoclassical age I do not know. But it seems plausible that in the complex of the doctor and the actor there exist discordant forces which comic theater could image in gest but could not expressly resolve. Argan's situation reveals that underlying social realities are manifest as a widespread uneasiness about where the foundations of character and human identity lie. The play employs Béralde and company and Purgon and their struggle for Argan's self as an immensely suggestive image of an endeavor to realize an ideal clarity and wholeness of self which elude human grasp. The agony here dramatized is doubly ironic: as Argan strives to gather together the scattered pieces of his selfhood, his struggle is repeatedly frustrated—not merely by the doctors, who are satirized ruthlessly, but also by the actors who in their own way violate the integrity of their patient.

By the end of the comedy Argan has distanced himself from the doctors and their follies and has escaped as well from the malignant scheming of Béline. In fact, however, all that he accomplishes is to exchange the earlier form of submissiveness for its analogue. The final riotous burlesque constitutes an ironic inversion of Argan's introductory, isolated monologue. In that dance Argan celebrates his freedom from the doctors' influence, but he does not see that he is now wholly subject to the communal will of the players with whom he dances. In this final scene Argan's identity is still visibly scripted: the only difference is that, whereas in the introductory scene his self was imprisoned, held rigid, now it whirls feverishly in the madness of the players' dance. Freed of the powers of the doctors, Argan now yields his self to the actors.

In the burlesque finale we see an Argan wholly different from the character who first took the stage yet one whose identity is just as tenuous. As initially he accepted the "text" of the doctors, so here, during his enthusiastic dance, he accepts the text of the actors. Argan exchanges the folly of the monomaniac for the enthusiasm of the celebrant. In so doing, he replaces an absolute resistance to change with an absolute flexibility. That is to say, he abandons medical "truth," which is illusory, and accepts the truth of the theater, which is illusion—which is, strictly speaking, the loss of self that constitutes madness:

> Entreé de Ballet
>
> Tous les Chirurgiens et Apothicaires viennent
> lui faire la révérence en cadence.
>
> **Bachelierus**
>
> > *Grandes doctores doctrinae*
> > *De la rhubarbe et du séné,*
> > *Ce serait sans douta à moi chosa folla,*
> > *Inepta et ridicula,*
> > *Si j'alloibam m'engageare*
> > *Vobis louangeas donare,*

Et entreprenoibam adjoutare
  Des lumieras au soleillo,
Et des étoilas au cielo,
  Des ondas à l'Oceano,
Et des rosas au printanno.
Agreate qu' avec uno moto,
  Pro toto remercimento,
Rendam gratiam corpori tam docto.
  Vobis, vobis debeo
Bien plus qu' à naturae et qu' à patri meo:
  Natura et pater meus
  Hominem me habent factum;
  Mais vos me, ce qui est bien plus,
  Avetis factum medicum,
  Honor, favor, et gratia
  Qui, in hoc corde que voilà,
  Imprimant ressentimenta
  Qui dureront in secula.

Chorus

Vivat, vivat, vivat, vivat, cent fois vivat,
  Novus Doctor, qui tam bene parlat!
Mille, mille annis et manget et bibat,
  Et seignet et tuat!

[Pp. 1176–77]

Obviously the audience derives great pleasure from this final frenzied extravaganza, and yet we would hesitate to call it a joyous spectacle. Neither is it socializing, unless by "socializing" we mean a process of communal scapegoating. The terms of Argan's integration with the community of actors are duplicitous, as duplicitous in their own way as was the promise of Dionysus to Pentheus. It is supremely ironic that Argan is once more obliged to fit his self into a text that others have written. When the play began he read from physicians' bills; here, at the very end of the comedy, he still obeys others' words: "But me? what am I to say, what am I to answer?" he asks Béralde (p. 1171).

As Béralde's answer indicates, even at this late date Argan remains powerless to invent his own text: "They will instruct you in a few words, and I will give you in writing what you must say.

Hurry and put on a decent outfit and I will send for them" (p. 1171). Significantly, at this point Angélique worries that her father will be made the butt of still more jokes: "But, uncle," she comments, "it appears to me that you are making too much fun of my father" (p. 1171). And Béralde's indirect reply—"it is only among ourselves" (p. 1171)—surely constitutes one of the play's most cryptic statements on the meaning of theatrical experience. The words are not a legitimate answer to Angélique's objection, just as the typical defense of certain slurs—I said it ("nigger," "hymie," "wop") in private conversation—constitutes no defense whatsoever. Angélique, for one, hardly seems reassured by Béralde's words, consenting to the performance only "since my uncle will direct us" (p. 1171).

Despite all the last-minute bustle, then, this moody scene ought not be overlooked. Readers especially tend to ignore Angélique's apprehensions because they come so near the end of the comedy, when the problems of the young lovers appear to have been solved. Yet the tone of these moments forms an eerie contrast with the clamor of the ensuing burlesque, and closer inspection reveals that Angélique's fears for her father's welfare are never fully allayed. Béralde maintains that "the carnival authorizes this" (p. 1171), but here, as elsewhere in this play, he does not speak for Molière, nor does his position fully express the emotional quality inherent in this moment. So we sometimes assure others of our own harmless intentions—it's all in play, it's all in jest—and yet Béralde's assurance rings counterfeit. His answer does not relieve Argan's fears; it simply rules them out of order. Argan has no choice: he *must* perform, *must* act out a fiction which someone else has written for him.

But what is even more unsettling about the conditions of Argan's final performance is the manner by which it is achieved. It comes in the guise of a subversive displacement, a displacement of identity which defines the problematic view of the theater inherent in this comedy. Argan does not simply change his mind with respect to his demand that Angélique marry a doctor; what happens is that Béralde and Toinette suddenly and completely usurp Argan's monomania and manipulate it to their ends:

BÉRALDE: But brother, an idea occurs to me: you become a doctor yourself. The convenience will be even greater, to have all that you need in yourself.
TOINETTE: That's true. There's the real way to cure yourself quickly; and there is no malady so bold, as to gamble with the person of a doctor.

[P. 1170]

Argan senses immediately that Béralde's motives are opaque, suspicious, and possibly hostile; he seems instinctively to perceive that his brother understands him in an unusually intrusive way—not in a rational sense, certainly, but psychically, as an actor, after long study of his part, may suddenly understand his role. Certainly Argan interprets Béralde's action as an ambivalent transgression of his self, and his response indicates his fear that that *self* has been objectified—"thinged"—preliminary to being incorporated into his brother's unknown plots. As he says, "I think, brother, that you are mocking me: am I of an age to be studying" (p. 1170)?

It is significant that Béralde answers Argan's second question but ignores the query implicit in his first statement: are you continuing to mock my fears? The conversation swiftly moves on, and so Béralde's motives remain largely mysterious. Whatever the source of his actions, the intimacy he displays here with respect to Argan constitutes a very real intrusion, and we may well doubt that it is entirely generous. In suddenly understanding his brother, Béralde in effect absorbs him: and Argan correctly perceives this displacement, this appropriation of self, to be taking place.

For members of the audience, Argan's nervousness is prelude to *sparagmos:* they interpret Béralde's suggestion as the empathic transgression it is. In these closing moments of the comedy Argan is exposed as a creature utterly without meaningful self, a disquieting manifestation of imagination's failure. To cure his suffering side, Argan was compelled to remove it from the power of the doctors and yield it to the power of the actors, but the play ends with no guarantee that what has once been torn to pieces can ever be made whole. Argan is funny because he cannot invent the language he needs for self-definition. His words—and so his identity—are always the exclusive, fashioned product of an Other. He reiterates a perpetual "Yes" to almost anyone who happens to be nearby and so comes dangerously close to selfless transparency. Strictly speaking, he acts the actor but from a new and quite modern perspective characterized primarily by an ironic fusion of theater and reality.

What, then, is the actor-audience paradigm which this play manifests? Certainly it is not possible to read this comedy in Bergsonian terms, as the affirmative conversion to health of the antisocial man. Neither is it possible to read the comedy only in terms of mythos, for it is not wholly "affirmative," "celebratory," or "redemptive," as those terms are frequently used to describe New Comedy.

In *Le malade imaginaire,* Molière lays bare Argan's paralyzing and ultimately irremediable condition: finally, he can be only what others want him to be. According to the theatrical vocabulary that this play requires its audience to adopt, we might summarize the condition thus: to be vital is to consent imaginatively to others, to be open to actorlike changes, and yet with freely given consent we inevitably acknowledge something which is its negation. Argan discovers in the course of the play that he can escape what terrifies him by feigning; he discovers that he can relieve his suffering by forsaking the doctors for the actors. But acting, too, denies him the integrity of self for which he so desperately yearns. Unless he acts, he cannot live successfully in the world, but once he begins to act he can fit into only a world of actors and must therefore conform to the world's notion of what he ought to be.

Molière thus writes comedy in which the theater functions simultaneously as a valid means to selfhood and as an ironic double deceit from which the self cannot escape. This quizzical perspective on theater makes *Le malade imaginaire* specially modern. At the center of this comedy is a model for comic theater which is to be reiterated endlessly during the modern period. Centuries later, the father in Pirandello's haunting *Six Characters in Search of an Author* expresses a subtext implicit in Molière's comedy, the terrible fact that a person may well be "nobody," in contrast to a character, who is always "somebody." "A character, sir," the father says, "may always ask a man who he is. Because a character has really a life of his own, marked with his especial characteristics." The identities of real people, in contrast, are evanescent fictions. The father questions the manager

> only in order to know if you, as you really are now, see yourself as you once were with all the illusions that were yours then, with all the things both inside and outside of you as they seemed to you—as they were then indeed for you. Well, sir, if you think of all those illusions that mean nothing to you now, of all those things which don't even *seem* to you to exist any more, while once they *were* for you, don't you feel that—I won't say these boards—but the very earth under your feet is sinking away from you when you reflect that in the same way this *you* as you feel it today—all this present reality of yours— is fated to seem a mere illusion to you tomorrow?[12]

So the self finds expression only in change, but to begin to change is inevitably to abandon all hope for lasting self-definition. The whole thrust of *Le malade imaginaire* is to transform Argan from one mask into another. He more fully develops the paradoxical gestus at the center of Molière's earlier farce on the same subject, *Le médecin malgré lui*. In that play, Sganarelle, the protagonist, is victimized by his wife's ingenious revenge. She convinces two men that her husband is a famous but exceedingly modest physician who needs to be coerced into admitting his professional expertise. The two strangers set upon the unsuspecting Sganarelle one day while he is in the forest cutting wood, and Sganarelle of course is unable to convince them that he knows nothing of medicine. Identity—not skill—is the issue. The men beat Sganarelle when he insists that he (and not they) truly knows who he is. The beatings hurt, and eventually, to avoid further pain, Sganarelle acknowledges that his tormentors know his identity better than he does. "Oh! oh! oh!" he wails; "Messieurs, I will be anything you please" (*Oeuvres,* 2, p. 236). He obligingly becomes a doctor. The new identity brings him immediate freedom from pain (and incidentally also brings wealth and sexual gratification), but these things are not obtained free of charge. By the end of the play Sganarelle is threatened with execution, and in order to save his life, he must recover his real self—which is precisely what Argan cannot do.

The hope that theater might be therapeutic has a long history on stage and in criticism, but *Le malade imaginaire* poses the familiar question of theater and therapy from an ironic standpoint. To see how it does so we might turn, finally, to the scene in which Toinette and Béralde persuade Argan to feign dying in order to discover which members of his family truly love him. The scene has a direct counterpart, of course, in Louison's playing dead, and it has analogues in most of the other previous instances of shamming. This is Argan's first obvious attempt at playing, however, and we must examine it carefully. The scene suggests that acting is something a person learns rather than purely a matter of natural ability. Argan expresses doubts about the performance. Significantly, he does not doubt his ability to act, but he questions the activity itself: he asks whether to counterfeit an action might not involve risks which the performer cannot see. His question is absolutely fascinating. Indeed, his perception of the condition of play has that uncanny simplicity and clarity associated conventionally with prophets or madmen: "Is there not any danger," he inquires gently, "in counterfeiting death?" (p. 1166).

Toinette, one of the chief representatives of the Others of the play, and thus someone for whom role playing is the "natural" way of life, assures Argan that everything may be feigned: "No, no: what danger can there be? Just stretch out. [*in a low voice*] It will be a pleasure to confuse your brother. Here is Madam. Hold on" (p. 1166).[13]

This scene, like so many in the play, raises laughter at Argan's expense. Even in reading we cannot help snickering at the hypochondriac's naivete. Yet Argan's question, despite its innocence, goes to the very core of the play. It is Molière's question, too, and the sound of laughter cannot completely lighten its gravity. As for the related question—does Toinette here speak for Molière?—the answer must be that she does not; she cannot (or will not) grasp Argan's anguish and pathos. Argan does not merely fear that playing dead, unlike playing doctor, is especially taboo. Perhaps, in his innocence, Argan worries that feigning an act might actually condemn him to live it, but more likely he fears playing dead for reasons which cannot be assigned to this or to any other simple rational cause. What Argan abandons with great reluctance is his overwhelming conviction that play is volatile and that to abandon personal fears in favor of an exterior model for self is to abandon something of great value with no guarantee that it will be returned. Argan perceives that to play any role, not simply this role, is to lose hold of individuality. He is afraid to mime dying not because he is concerned that counterfeit action will invoke reality but because he knows intuitively that to give one's self over to the Other is, in a very real sense, to die.

Like Sganarelle, Argan is forced to adopt a hypocritical existence. Indeed what choice does either have? But does it then make sense to attribute free choice to Louison? or to Toinette? or to Angélique? It makes little difference that both these plays are comedies, just as it makes little difference that both Sganarelle and Argan are technically improved by the operations of the Others if by "improvement" we mean that they are made to "fit" better into society. The price of such socializing is great indeed—and its value, ultimately, is moot. Without acting, a person exists in pain; but acting in turn is a trap from which there is no escape. Once we start to act, we surrender any claim to an original selfhood. The *acting* constitutes the identity.

Finally, then, the obvious questions: if nothing cannot be simulated, to what extent does simulation routinely contaminate everyday life? Do people act in private as well as in public? Is the world indeed a theater? And is someone deceiving someone else on every occasion? When, then, are children children? When are illnesses real? When is one's self one's own, or is this "I" merely the fictitious product of institutionally sustained belief? And are even the dead—we may recall the spooky words of Molière's epitaph (which is of course a sham epitaph)—also playing a role?

More recent comic playwrights sometimes pose these questions explicitly and brutally. Harold Pinter, for example, asks in much the same way about the rights of self and the rights of Others in *The Birthday Party.* The subject is important to Brecht, too. Galy Gay, the protagonist of Brecht's mocking comedy of the selfless self, *Mann ist Mann,* forsakes an ineffectual self which is uniquely *his* for the vitalizing and ironically triumphant flux of an identity tailored by others. Gay, like Argan, is dismantled and rebuilt like a piece of machinery. In the case of Galy Gay we discover a comedy whose happy ending is keenly ironic. Gay purchases happiness (or worldly success, its apparent substitute) by obligingly becoming anything the other soliders want him to be. As with Argan, however, such flexibility proves to be its own kind of fixity. Likewise, if we follow *Le malade imaginaire* to its center, we discover in it an almost Jansenist core, a profoundly moving contemplation of the possibility that existence is nothing more than a piece of theater and that human individuality may prove to be a vain fiction— simply a relative matter.[14] Brecht states the case more bluntly than Molière—"People who talk about 'personality' can kiss my ass"[15]—but both playwrights nevertheless reach the same conclusion.

For earlier comic playwrights, feigning was sometimes the precursor to genuine growth. We may recall, say, Gonzalo's recitation of the curative metamorphoses wrought on Prospero's magic island, "when no man was his own" (*The Tempest,* V.i.213). But the gestural connotations of Molière's comedy are entirely different, and by looking first backward to earlier Renaissance works and then forward to modern theater, we can see that *Le malade imaginaire* anticipates a shift in emphasis which characterizes much modern drama. From beginning to end, Argan can only live out others' scripts. Molière is the first important creator of comic theater to write plays which take on meaning not because the hero *becomes* an actor, as did the heroes of many earlier playwrights, but because an actor is already in some ironic sense the play's hero.

PART III
Modern Models

Seventeenth-century playwrights have proved fundamental in shaping modern notions of comedy, and when we think about more recent comic theaters the inevitable tendency is to place them with respect to something loosely defined as *the* comic tradition. As a result some writers are inevitably "wrong" about comedy, while others are "right," and ultimately unsatisfactory debates take place as to which of several writers is "most traditional" or most "comic." The limitations inherent in the concept of a Darwinian literary tradition have often been noted, and yet the concept of a continuing cultural effort so powerfully grips the mind that it sometimes blinds us—to use Emerson's phrase for it—to the fact that we too enjoy an original relation with the universe. It is possible, for example, to argue for a tradition of English mannered comedy that extends backward from Harold Pinter through Somerset Maugham and Arthur Wing Pinero and Edward Bulwer-Lytton and the George Colmans to the playwrights of the Restoration stage, thence even further back through Jonson and Plautus and the dramatists who composed Greek New Comedy. Doubtless it makes sense to speak of versions or variants of mannered comedy. But we cannot proceed to assume that a contemporary comic dramatist will be interested only in dramatizing stories or themes similar to those that interested Menander or Jonson.

The temptation in looking at older comic theaters is to view them in terms of modern concepts of theatricality, making something which was once provocative and sometimes threatening into something harmless, furry, or cute and then equating *those* meanings with the comic "truth." We must not minimize the capacity of older societies to shape comedy according to specific contemporary needs; neither must we minimize the potential of modern comic theaters to respond to realities which prove as troubling as society's progressive theatricalization proved to be for seventeenth-century audiences. There have been many important comic theaters since those of Jonson and Molière, and the playwrights who created such theaters have attempted more than the updating of old scripts. Most of them offer new metaphors to define the nature of the actor's relationship with his audience. In the final sequence of essays in this book I want to discuss two of the best and most significant examples of modern comic theaters.

5 *The Cherry Orchard:* Text Versus Performance

> Vaudeville-plots abound in me as does oil
> in the depths of Baku.
> —Anton Chekhov, letter to
> A. S. Souvorin, December 23, 1888

Chekhov's plays are sometimes thought to lack genre despite much evidence from his many letters that he wrote with great sensitivity to the particular kind of work he was creating.[1] *Three Sisters* was called a "drama," a term which for Chekhov identified specific generic characteristics, while *The Sea Gull* and *The Cherry Orchard* were termed "comedies." As people who write about Chekhov's theater habitually observe, Stanislavsky's melancholy interpretations at the Moscow Art Theatre caused the playwright much irritation and even despair. Especially upsetting to Chekhov was Stanislavsky's production of *The Cherry Orchard,* which the author called "the undoing of my play."[2] If Stanislavsky's productions accomplished nothing else, however, they proved that Chekhov's works, and especially *The Cherry Orchard,* can be performed successfully according to a wide variety of styles, and it is now possible to speak of several distinct Chekhovian performance traditions, ranging from pathetic to prophetic to farcical.[3] Doubtless all truly great dramatic texts are open to reinterpretation; still, we cannot infer that there is no value in attempting to understand Chekhov's theater as he himself conceived it—that is, as an exploration of histrionic possibilities which "comedy" suggested to the playwright.[4]

Consider the introductory sequence of events in *The Cherry Orchard:*

The Cherry Orchard: Act One

A room that still goes by the name of the nursery. One of the doors leads up to Anya's room. It is dawn and the sun will soon come up. It is May. The cherry trees are in flower, but in the orchard it is cold, there is morning frost. The windows in the room are closed. Enter Dunyasha *with a candle and* Lopakhin *with a book in his hand.*

LOPAKHIN. The train's arrived, thank the Lord. What's the time?

DUNYASHA. Almost two o'clock. [*Extinguishes the candle.*] It's already light.

LOPAKHIN. How late was the train, how many hours? About two at least. [*Yawns and stretches himself.*] Of all the stupid tricks to pull, damned if I haven't gone and done it again. I came here on purpose so I could meet them at the station, and before you know it, I slept right through it . . . Went dead to sleep sitting up. Annoying, that's what . . . If only you might've awakened me.

DUNYASHA. I thought you'd left. [*Listens.*] There, I think they're coming now.

LOPAKHIN. [*Listens.*] No . . . they've got luggage to get, and one thing or another . . . [*Pause.*] Lyubov Andreevna has been living five years abroad, and I don't know what she's become now . . . She's a very fine person. An obliging person, simple. I remember when I was a youngster about fifteen, my father—he's dead now but at the time he was a shopkeeper in the village here—hit me in the face with his fist. The blood ran out of my nose . . . We had come to the yard here for some reason, and he'd been drinking. Lyubov Andreevna, as I remember right now, was still very young, such a slim woman she was. She led me over to the washstand here in this very room, the nursery. "Don't cry, little peasant," she says "it will heal before your wedding . . ." [*Pause.*] Little peasant . . . It's true my father was a peasant, and here I am in a white waistcoat and yellow boots. Like a pig's nozzle showing up in a row of wedding cakes . . . It's just that I'm rich, lots of money for sure, but if you really think about it and look into it, you'll know I'm just a peasant through and through . . . [*Turns the pages of the book.*] I read this book and didn't catch on to a single thing. I was reading and fell right to sleep. [*Pause.*]

[Pp. 165–66]

For many years this and similar Chekhovian scenes have been praised for their apparent fidelity to the ragged texture of real life. In fact, however, there is no reason to assume that Chekhov's realism is any less problematic than the realistic visual arts of other ages. As E. H. Gombrich has shown, realism in art is always historically and culturally conditioned, so that what seems "true to life" in one period appears consciously stylized when measured by the standards of any other.[5] It cannot be demonstrated that this drama is more faithful to reality than that of many other theaters, ancient or modern; these days, as a matter of interest, Chekhovian comedy seems a good deal less realistic in performance than, say, that of Harold Pinter. But we *can* show that this scene disrupts a modern theatrical frame according to which a player who appears on stage is expected to remain "in character." For example, Lopakhin especially exhibits an eerie rationality because of the way his words apply simultaneously to player and role. When he discusses his clothes and his book, his acting style is neither lifelike nor artificial but—within the representational frame—almost hallucinatory. He starts to deliver a piece of exposition, pauses, drifts, starts again, then comments self-consciously about a book he is holding. The words of Lopakhin (the fiction) correspond oddly to the gestural reality of the player; these words are not sufficiently detached to constitute an objective commentary on the performer or his play, as they sometimes do in Brechtian performances, and yet they establish a provocative resonance between actor and character. Lopakhin exhibits a mode of behavior in which one is both leading and being led, placing one foot in front of the other, as it were, cautiously but unwittingly. The result is a seamless behavioral mode which is both subjective and investigative: an approach to character, or an exploration of the topography of character, rather than a straightforward naturalistic representation.

In this chapter I shall examine the histrionic structure of *The Cherry Orchard* in order to see to what extent a new orientation of performer and role can give the illusion of a new genre. My discussion will center on the quality of the actors' ensemble performance, and on the cooperative interactions of players and audience in the production of Chekhovian comedy.

One of the most revealing facts about the composition of *The Cherry Orchard* is its relationship to the then popular "mortgage" melodrama. In his study of modern drama, *The Theater of Revolt*, Robert Brustein summarizes the differences between *The Cherry Orchard* and a typical play done in the manner of conventional melodramas, Dion Boucicault's *The Octoroon:* "The gentle victim (Mrs. Peyton) becomes the irresponsible and self-destructive Lyuba Ranevsky; the virtuous low-born ingenue (Zoe) becomes the weepy, nunlike Varya; the humorous friend (Salem Scudder) becomes the indigent buffoon, Pishtchik; the pathetic old servant (Pete) becomes the comically senile Firs; and the moustache-twirling villain (McCloskey) becomes the generous and warmhearted Lopakhin."[6] As Brustein notes, in each case Chekhov overturns the melodramatic formula, reversing its conventions partly to satirize them and partly to take ironic advantage of spectators' expectations.

In moving his characters away from melodrama, however, Chekhov does not move them toward "real life." If anything, he enhances their "staginess" by caricaturing each according to a particular affective outline. The gentle victim of melodrama becomes an obvious poseur; the humble ingenue becomes a crybaby; age becomes senility, and humor, buffoonery. Most of the changes shift the roles decisively toward farce: buffoon, *senex,* virgin, and so on. These familiar comic roles define the generic potential of the play; insofar as spectators detect them, they constitute the comic "horizon of expectations."[7] *The Cherry Orchard* evokes antecedent farcical texts. But the familiar outlines are only decoys: the farce is rendered problematic by a performance style that partly subverts the production of a "farcical" text. In particular, the anticipated aggressive energy one expects of the farce ensemble never quite materializes. The result for an audience is the illusion not of real life but of "failed" comic theater, an altogether different experience.

Let me clarify my position. Most studies of Chekhov take a representational approach; they ignore the actor in the belief that Chekhov wrote theater that wholly absorbed spectators in the fiction unrolling before their eyes. But an awareness of the actors acting is an important component of Chekhov's comic theater. Granted, Chekhov's actors do not conspicuously acknowledge their play, as did those of Aristophanes or Plautus. But they nevertheless manifest a characteristic response *to* that play. That response constitutes the basic gest of the comedy: to act *The Cherry Orchard* successfully, Chekhov's actors must somehow persuade the audience of their essential inadequacy to mount a farce. The actors' comedic performance must visibly falter at certain crucial moments, creating for an audience a comic theater whose meaning ironically lays bare the futility and the inappropriateness of the histrionic gestures which people make to each other and to the world.

There is a difference, after all, between telling an actor to "live the part" or to "live the life." The latter method results normally in a uniformly "depressed" performance style such as is common in film or television. But such a style seems not to have accorded with Chekhov's own ambitions for his comedy. To be sure, Chekhov always labored during rehearsals to correct actors who overacted. Yet Chekhov's demands on his actors were quite paradoxical and could not be achieved by actors who simply pretended not to be acting at all.[8] The actors who play in *The Cherry Orchard* must *act*, of course; in addition, however, they must find a way occasionally to mask the "irrepressibility" component of conventional farce.[9] One way to disguise the familiar aggressiveness that signifies "farce" to an onlooker is to place it under apparent stress, so that the spectators grow less conscious that they are in the presence of a fully rehearsed performance regulated by a script. A crude analogy would be the circus acrobat who deliberately fails in his act once or twice before achieving success. Similarly, if an actor in a farce occasionally and apparently accidentally retards his gestural style, the audience will sense that something unknown is threatening the production of the script, which should appear to be effortless. In this case the actor's random "disabilities" redirect spectators' attentions to the affective framework of his art. If such maneuvers intrude upon the farce only irregularly, they cannot be perceived by onlookers as scripted; if anything, they seem distinctly ambiguous.

Hence the characteristic baffling and often irritating performance style of *The Cherry Orchard:* the slightly mistimed responses, the inappropriate gestures, the awkward pauses and contradictory emotional rhythms must seem to be the work of an ensemble straining—and just barely failing—to achieve a successful "comic" performance. The actors' communal "failure" to produce the comic text then becomes the basis of the play's histrionic power. These secretly scripted failings disengage the actors from their farcical masks. More important, they make the actors' playing quite disorienting for an audience to behold. Instead of permitting spectators to experience the familiar energies of vaudeville or farce, Chekhov's actors stage a performance provocatively unpleasant. Their playing provides a renewed experience of comedy which includes chagrin, even psychic pain; the play gives the impression of moving beyond or through comedy further than we supposed possible. Alternatively, we could say that Chekhov develops a theater in which "comedy" is itself an important element of the performance: the players seize the familiar vaudeville masks but seem unable to manage sufficient energy to keep the world of their play intact.

The histrionic force of *The Cherry Orchard,* then, does not depend entirely on Chekhov's humanizing the farcical outlines of his characters. It derives as well from the ability of the actors to make it clear to an audience that the familiar roles are being played in an unfamiliar style. Chekhov repeatedly centers his comedy on a single recurring gest—a speaker who fails through some inherent weakness to hold the attention of his audience or to create the effect he desires with respect to his onlookers. Each actor/character is at some level a humorous type who attempts repeatedly to dominate the stage with his or her particular humorous mechanism or eccentricity: weeping, time keeping, a hearing deficiency, billiards, cards, a stock phrase, or a nervous tic. But in some peculiar way all these individual performances lack their customary jack-in-the-box vitality, so that the irrepressible energy which we expect to characterize the farcical performance always issues stillborn.

A useful comparison may be drawn here between the histrionic force of *The Cherry Orchard* and *Bartholomew Fair.* In each case the playwright assigns most of the characters a "humorous" personality and then arranges the action in terms of the competing and often alien interests. Chekhov is always filling the stage, as did Jonson, with crowds of actors who clamor for the audience's attention: in *The Cherry Orchard,* as in *Bartholomew Fair,* scenes of half a dozen or more actors are common, and surprise entrances are frequent. Yet the effect which Chekhov achieves is quite the opposite of what we naturally expect of such potentially farcical encounters. His crowd scenes lack the anticipated comic vitality; instead, we repeatedly confront a group of would-be comedians whose play is disturbingly inadequate, and we are never sure that the performance will not collapse entirely.

The unspecified uneasiness characteristic of a "successful" performance of *The Cherry Orchard* is psychologically kin to the dismay audiences feel when any performance, whether play or sporting event or lion-taming act, unexpectedly begins to break up. Chekhov's strange pauses, the unanticipated changes in mood or in rhythm, the famous breaking string, all are perceived as threats to the integrity of the script; they are textural gaps through which "reality" intrudes upon the performance. Watching *The Cherry Orchard* is sometimes like watching an actor who is playing Macbeth (for example) forget his lines. Suddenly the familiar "scriptedness" vanishes, and the result is embarrassment and usually sympathy for the performer. Spectators who may have assumed that they were uninvolved bystanders suddenly lose their sense of detachment in a heteropathic surge of feeling—for the player, not for the persona. They yearn to act—that is, to help—yet they are permitted to do nothing. All at once they lose the organizational safety net which the modern theatrical frame provides on the staged events, and they find themselves in the uncomfortable position of having no clear role to play. The inevitable consequence is nervousness or —ncreased tension. Even fear and anger are not uncommon in situations when the performance threatens to dissolve. With these considerations in mind, we can now shift the discussion of Chekhov's comedy into a more specific analysis, one which will illuminate the relationship of play to public.

Let us return to the introductory scene of *The Cherry Orchard* to consider in greater detail its affective structure. In the proscenium arch theater, the raising of the curtain brackets the ensuing events. The rising curtain defines the magical "fourth wall": it signals to the onlookers in the darkened auditorium that they may now assume their roles as unseen watchers and opens the imitated world to their privileged eyes. It signals also that the actors will collaborate with the expectations of the audience in the presentation of the fiction. When an actor first appears, he or she will pretend not to be aware of the observers. The actors may alter their physical stances when speaking to one another so as to reveal the dynamics of their interactions, and they may even stare occasionally into the darkness that lies beyond the edge of the stage. But their eyes never acknowledge the gaze of the spectators. Even during the performance of a comedy, which necessitates frequent pauses in the dialogue to provide space for the audience to laugh, that "acknowledgment" constitutes no acknowledgment. The play may be melodramatic or naturalistic, stagey or low key. Whatever the mode or performance style, however, the representational frame demands that the actors always be "in character." And within this context the effect of even farcical performances depends on the actors' playing their roles in as straightforward a manner as possible.[10]

Such, then, are the basic, typical expectations of audiences of the early modern period. For an audience accustomed to this particular theatrical frame, the introductory moments of *The Cherry Orchard* prove severely disruptive. The first events of the comedy consist in great measure of lazy waiting: the lead actor pauses, yawns, and utters an introductory speech that seems to include much irrelevant commentary. Lopakhin delivers a more-or-less straightforward expository narrative, but the rhythm of his diction is at odds with a performance that audiences will interpret theatrically as "natural." Realism (as a movement) in the theater demands that the player produce his discourse without apparent histrionic effort, but Lopakhin speaks in a manner which partly opens that effort to view. This effect is achieved primarily by means of the unanticipated pauses which interrupt the exposition: "Lyubov Andreevna has been living five years abroad, and I don't know what she's become now . . . She's a very fine person. An obliging person, simple. I remember when I was a youngster about fifteen, my father—he's dead now but at the time he was a shopkeeper in the village here—hit me in the face with his fist" (p. 166).

In the lengthy silences that pall the atmosphere of this first scene of *The Cherry Orchard,* we glimpse an actor dimly visible behind his mask. Any theatergoer grasps instantly that Lopakhin's role is functional: he must swiftly take charge of the stage and deliver an informational speech. But Lopakhin offers an audience the necessary orientation in a disorienting manner. Lopakhin's behavior radically departs from the probable expectations of Chekhov's audience, not only because of his faltering delivery, but also because his commentary seems peculiarly self-conscious. It is as if "acting" acquires both its connotations simultaneously: "doing" and "seeming to do." Persona and personality play off against one another like a set of opposed mirrors. The actor/character comments obliquely on his costume: "and here I am in a white waistcoat and yellow boots. Like a pig's nozzle showing up in a row of wedding cakes." Next he fiddles with a book hitherto unattended by spectators: "[*Turns the pages of the book.*] I read this book and didn't catch on to a single thing. I was reading and fell right to sleep. [*Pause.*]" (p. 166). Following this last remark, the stage again falls silent. Two, three, possibly more seconds pass, as indicated by the stage direction, and on that flattened note, Chekhov concludes the initial beat of his comedy.

It is an astonishing introductory sequence. During a few short minutes of playing time Chekhov effectively dislodges the audience from its accustomed representational frame. Because of the manner in which the staged representation spirals insistently back into the representing, the onlookers cannot follow Lopakhin or Dunyasha by means of any familiar affective or cognitive structure. The silences alone will not permit them to engage the play as they normally would. The pauses deny spectators the passive involvement with conventionally energetic figures on a realistic stage. As a result, they are likely to be confused, even upset; and in their confusion and anxiety they cannot help but become involved with the reality of the Figuren whom they see before them. Where they expect conventional (in the sense that it is capable of passing unnoticed) histrionic power, Chekhov substitutes apparent impotence; and the actors' disturbing lassitude compels a powerful, albeit unfocused, response on the part of the audience, which is required somehow to supply the psychic energy to complete the obviously "inadequate" performance.

The result is that Chekhov writes a participatory comedy, though not in any ritualistic or therapeutic sense nor, indeed, in Stanislavsky's sense that the text encourages spectators to reconstruct the emotional history of the individual characters. Rather the audience is here encouraged to join with the ensemble in uncovering and redefining the meaning of the entire theater event. The tension and nervousness characteristic of Chekhov's comedy is born of the spectators' knowledge that they are deeply implicated in the actors' play yet are powerless to will its success. At the center of the comedy is the paradox of "realistic" theater which permits spectators to weep at the death of the persona (if it is performed zealously) but not to engage the actors in any direct way. This paradox makes Chekhov's comedy so radically different from anything that precedes it. It also makes the drama deeply troubling, "tragicomic," to use the word most frequently associated with the typical Chekhovian atmosphere. If the comic actors seem unable to maintain the energy necessary to protect their play world from an exterior reality, how can the audience fail to be perplexed, upset, even grieved? The players' illusion is of a body of information—a text—which has not been sufficiently assimilated, and the price such theater exacts from its audience is extremely high. Spectators' suffering is not only an empathetic sharing of the characters' fictional agonies but also a particular yearning for the reassurance provided by a scripted histrionic performance.

During the lengthy pause which follows Lopakhin's speech, the only sounds are those of the theater—those which are normally not heeded during a realistic performance.[11] Spectators are forced, therefore, to listen to the superior reality beyond the performance. Depending on the length of the actors' pauses in their speech, the silence may grow distinctly uncomfortable for onlookers. Audiences at the turn of the century were unused to such silences on the stage, and the effect was profoundly disorienting, even spooky. It was like being made suddenly to concentrate on the spaces between the words of a speaker, which are always felt but are normally ignored as meaningless. For example, at the moment when Lopakhin fiddles with his book, visible histrionic endeavor reaches an embarrassingly still point. As the seconds pass, the audience yearns for the "play" to continue. At last Dunyasha speaks, but her words come as a surprise. In the context of the previous silence, her words take on, because of their suddenness, the felt quality of noise; thus they play off against the inevitable real noises of the theater: chairs squeaking, spectators' breathing, the occasional cough. In addition their content initiates a line of thought radically different from the previous one. It sounds almost as if Dunyasha were handing Lopakhin a lost thread of the dialogue: "The dogs didn't sleep the whole night. They can sense their masters are coming" (p. 166).

Oddly, however, this remark remains unanswered, and Lopakhin's silence only emphasizes the bizarre context of Dunyasha's speech. Her words echo, as if spoken down a well. They are linked with nothing before and institute no new direction in the conversation. Lopakhin seems not to hear them or not to understand. As silence once more envelops the stage, spectators again sense their enormous emotional investment in the actors' play. The play reaches a second histrionic crisis, so to speak, and the accumulated emotion of the moment finds its expression in a gestural emblem of imminent histrionic collapse:

> LOPAKHIN. What is it with you, Dunyasha, such . . .
> DUNYASHA. My hands are shaking. I'm going to faint.
> LOPAKHIN. You're really delicate, Dunyasha, too much so. You dress yourself like a lady, and your hair is fixed up the same way. You can't do things like that. Better remember who you are.
>
> [P. 166]

Now Lopakhin attempts to keep the performance under way, ministering to an actress who seems to hover on the brink of nervous failure. Dunyasha's nervousness opens to view the gestural realm of *The Cherry Orchard*. She manifests what in the comedy will become a social gestus, a person trying and failing to act the part he or she wants to play. Dunyasha's nervousness is focused upon, made readable for spectators. In conjunction with Lopakhin's self-reflexive commentary it exposes a whole network of essentially fraudulent relationships: player to persona, performer to spectator, the "real life" playing of roles, and so on. Dunyasha here becomes a "speaking picture" which manifests the essential falsity of histrionic endeavor. Theatrical illusion is refracted into its primal components, and the integrity of the play world, the hallmark of representational theater, begins to break down.

As if in response to this threat to the play world, Yepikhodov enters, behaving like a buffoon. Here, too, dramatic form follows from the psychology of the audience. The introductory sequence has so disrupted the representational frame that theatergoers are caught short. They are in danger of breaking frame entirely. By the time that Dunyasha threatens to faint, the silences have been too many. For an audience not familiar with this kind of performance, whispers, laughter, even hooting are real possibilities. Yepikhodov's unexpected entrance organizes the spectators' inchoate energy so that it will not issue, say, in catcalls and so demolish the performance. Of particular interest are Chekhov's stage directions which cover Yepikhodov's entrance: "YEPIKHODOV enters, carrying a bouquet. He wears a jacket and brightly scrubbed high boots that squeak loudly. Entering, he drops the bouquet" (p. 166). Yepikhodov's entrance comes when the audience is highly tensed, and it immediately releases that tension in a burst of laughter. J. L. Styan notes that Yepikhodov's "laughable appearance immediately uplifts the play."[12] Indeed it does, or it seems to. Perhaps the onlookers do not fully comprehend why Yepikhodov's sudden appearance is so funny—in performance there is scarcely time to fathom complex emotional responses—but they greet this new character with an enormous sense of relief.

Note that audiences do not laugh at Yepikhodov only because he *represents* a funny man. The onlookers' laughter here is nervous, wrought first of their own suppressed tension and next of their sudden perception of the particular quality of Yepikhodov's performance. His entrance gives the impression of a series of accidents *on the part of the actor who is playing him.* And spectators' laughter has a further distinguishing characteristic: it is not at first possible for them to say whether they are laughing at a scripted piece of buffoonery or at a genuine failure on the part of the actor. They respond here, in other words, as spectators *and* as theatergoers. The laughter is not merely cathartic but educative too, as if they exhaled in collective understanding: Ah, so it is to be a comedy of bad acting![13] Audiences laugh at Yepikhodov (and clearly they must) because they know that squeaky boots ought to have been oiled before the performance and that competent actors do not drop flowers which they are supposed to convey across the stage. Their response to Yepikhodov, in other words, is in the same mode as previous responses to Dunyasha and Lopakhin. In both instances they respond to actors who seem in danger of losing command of their play.

Buffoonery soon gives way to a third variation of "failed" histrionics. The scene involving Yepikhodov diverts spectators' attentions away from the homecoming, so that the arrival of Lyubov Andreevna and her retinue comes as a surprise. Within moments the stage swarms with people that onlookers cannot differentiate. Dunyasha the fiction proves to be an inept servant as well as an inept expositor: instead of announcing her mistress's arrival, she threatens to faint. Dunyasha and Lopakhin exit, the stage is empty for some moments, and then is heard the noise of a group of actors off stage.

>   DUNYASHA. [*agitated*] I'm going to faint right now. . . .
>   Oh, I know I'm going to faint!
>   *Two carriages are heard driving up to the house.* Lopakhin *and* Dunyasha *quickly go out. The stage is empty. The sound of hubbub begins in the adjoining rooms. Leaning on a stick,* Firs *hurriedly goes across the stage. He has been to the station to meet* Lyubov Andreevna. *He wears old-fashioned livery and a high hat. He keeps saying something to himself, but not a single word can be understood. The noise offstage keeps growing louder. A voice is heard saying:* "Let's go through here." *Enter, all walking through the room,* Lyubov Andreevna, Anya, *and* Sharlotta Ivanova *with a small*

dog on a chain—all are in traveling clothes—Varya, *wearing an overcoat and a scarf over her head,* Gaev, Simeonov-Pischik, Lopakhin, Dunyasha *with a bundle and an umbrella, and servants with luggage.*

[P. 167]

This is no ordinary arrival of characters on stage, and its peculiarly disorienting effect should not be ignored. Governing it are the same techniques which structured the introductory scene: actors who seem to be performing on the edge of error. Firs, for example, the first person to inhabit the empty stage, mumbles words which an audience cannot hear—though, lacking the text before them, they must assume that they are meant to. When audible conversation finally begins, there are too many characters on stage for them all to hold a conversation, and so the actors break into smaller groups, each with its own separate topic and separate style. In the theater the splitting tends initially to be disorienting, particularly since no protagonist emerges to focus spectators' attentions. In one area of the stage, Lyubov Andreevna, weeping, addresses Varya and her brother, nearly overcome with emotion; meanwhile Gaev, apparently embarrassed, partly detaches himself from the conversation and comments about inefficient rail service. Sharlotta and Pischik have formed a second conversational center, their irrelevant commentary undercutting spectators' empathetic involvement with the homecoming:

SHARLOTTA. [*to* Pischik] My dog eats nuts, too.
PISCHIK. [*surprised*] What do you think of that!

[P. 168]

Meanwhile, Dunyasha and Anya have drawn together, as if in preparation for an important scene: everyone else exits, leaving the two women alone on the stage. Dunyasha indeed attempts to tell Anya important news, but Anya—in another of the many scenes in *The Cherry Orchard* in which an auditor does not respond in the expected manner to a speaker—ignores her. Dunyasha is eager to tell Anya of Yepikhodov's proposal, but Anya will not listen: she responds "listlessly" (p. 168) to the excited Dunyasha, interrupting the tale of romance with idle commentary about lost hairpins, her old room, the rigors of travel.

The Cherry Orchard 139

Scenes involving actor/characters who cannot meaningfully connect with their onstage audiences are plentiful in *The Cherry Orchard*. The single most important gestural configuration in the comedy, it defines visually an ironic discord between a central Figur and one or more observers. Everyone remembers the most noticeable dramatizations of noncommunication in Chekhov: the skewed dialogue, the pauses, the deadend or irrelevant remarks. These, however, are verbal configurations of the basic gest of the comedy. At the end of Act I, for example, Varya's discourse lulls Anya to sleep, while somewhat earlier Pishchik does the same thing to himself: "And my Dashenka . . . keeps saying also that . . . she keeps saying all sorts of words. [*Snores, but immediately wakes up.*] Be that as it may, my honored lady, if you'll oblige me with . . . a loan of two hundred and forty rubles . . . I can pay the interest due on the mortgage tomorrow" (p. 175).

Too, the old manservant Firs, because he is deaf, recreates wherever he goes illusions of failed performances; whenever he asks someone to repeat himself, he is, in effect, asking that actor/character to project his voice with more authority. And when, in one of the play's most poignant moments, Gaev speaks eloquently to the bookcase, the embarrassment an offstage audience feels clearly depends upon his recognition that he has embarrassed his onstage listeners.

In focusing upon characters who cannot connect with their auditors in the manner in which they desire, Chekhov creates a series of onstage encounters between actors and audiences which shape the responses of the real audience offstage. Wherever we turn, we encounter characters who in one way or another are always embarrassing the people who attend them, or are boring them or even putting them to sleep. By requiring his actors to act the parts of failed comedians, Chekhov was able to develop a model for comedy in which the received forms of older theaters were the materials for innovative creation.

If we remember that comedies of most eras carry for their audiences powerful charges of fear, then Chekhov's comedy clearly cannot arbitrarily be isolated from earlier forms of comic theater merely because it elicits ambivalent responses from spectators. The basis of Chekhov's comedy is a very carefully modulated rhythm of performance: it is no more a "realistic" theater than, say, Ernest Hemingway's dialogue is a realistic rendering of the way people talk. Chekhov in fact creates a highly stylized comedy, one whose performance rhythms are syncopative. The effect is to create what Charles Timmer some years ago called "mental airpockets": gaps, pauses, embarrassing lapses when "one gasps for breath, until the tension is relieved by laughter."[14] The performance calls upon the actors to make an absurd remark at the "wrong" time, or an inappropriate gesture at the most "inappropriate" moment, or to act in what the audience will perceive to be an incongruous style. In performance, Chekhov's most characteristic effect is to irritate an audience—at least an audience that expects familiar genres or conventionally representational productions. Hence the strange and disquieting histrionic force which these plays can sometimes achieve: we measure the life of any theatrical performance by its rhythms of change. In the delicate and exquisitely *"mistimed"* rhythms of *The Cherry Orchard,* we witness the consequences when the apparent failure of the script forever lets the "real world" intrude upon the world of the play. Chekhov's plays are always in danger of dissolving into reality, with the result that this comedy—one of the high points of the modern comic theater—explores the relationship between stage and society in an elliptical and highly ironic manner.

The most meaningful moments in *The Cherry Orchard* tend to be those moments when the actors' play is most seriously threatened with disaster, when, as in Act I, we sense the actors buckling under the weight of an exterior reality that their comedic effort seems unable to withstand. It is no accident that the most intense moment of theater in all Chekhov—the celebrated breaking string which is heard twice in *The Cherry Orchard*—constitutes an intrusion from *beyond* the stage. "To interpret that sound," as Styan argues, "is to interpret the play."[15] Enigmatic, dying slowly away, the sound is infinitely suggestive, and yet it cannot be read strictly as a literary symbol, the emblem of hope or change or the passing of an order. It has great histrionic value, too. With it

Chekhov sums up the essential experience of his theater, which is always enacting, as it were, a dying fall. The sound comes from somewhere outside the play world, outside the sphere, that is, over which the actors may visibly exercise control. It signifies nothing less (and, in performance, nothing more!) than a momentary threat to the integrity of their playing.

Ultimately, the breaking string accords with the whole design of Chekhov's play. In that melancholy intrusion lies the essence of Chekhov's comic theater. The two occasions on which the string sounds yield additional information about the playwright's art. The sound first occurs in Act II, which is set in a field not far from the border of the orchard. Here, as elsewhere, Chekhov first leads his audience to the point at which the performance begins to falter; Gaev has just delivered another poorly timed speech, embarrassing the people who surround him both onstage and offstage and provoking another minor crisis in the production of the script:

> GAEV. [*in a low voice, as if reciting*] Oh, nature, marvelous nature, shining with eternal radiance, beautiful yet unfeeling, you whom we name as mother, in whom are united both the living and the dead, you give life and you destroy . . .
> VARYA. [*beseechingly*] Uncle dear!
> ANYA. Uncle, you're starting again!
> TROFIMOV. You'd better try a bank shot off the yellow into the middle.
> GAEV. I'll keep silent, silent.
> *All are sitting, deep in thought. Silence. All that can be heard is* Firs, *who mumbles quietly. Suddenly a sound is heard far off in the distance, as if coming from the sky. It is the sound of a string breaking that dies away sadly.*
> [P. 188]

That sound is as fearful to the audience as it is to the characters (and its effect in performance is truly shocking) because, hearing it, spectators realize how desperate is their need to believe in the integrity of the actors' play and in their own superior reality. Once again, the players' odd quiescence creates a vacuum in the play world, and the inevitable consequence is that reality enters by way of the subtext. It is commonplace to observe that the sound of the breaking string ruptures the so-called dramatic illusion, but in the particular context of *The Cherry Orchard,* that event is but one of many instances which cause the audience to experience what Jean Piaget might describe as a forced accommodation to reality.[16] The consummatory hopes of audience and players are suddenly threatened by an intrusion from beyond the play world—from a realm, that is, against which no script can ever guard. In consequence, an audience is forced to integrate its experience of the actors' play with something larger, something more vital, something hostile which threatens to tear it apart.

The second time the string sounds, its menace is even more pronounced. Chekhov prepares his audience for this moment very carefully. Just before the end of the play, all the characters depart; the stage grows empty, and all that is heard are sounds offstage: doors being locked, carriages driving away, the first blows of the axes. This sound, Chekhov says, is "solitary and dolorous" (p. 210), and the play seems over. Suddenly there are footsteps, and through a door on the right shuffles Firs, apparently ill. He goes to an exterior door and touches its handle. He then discovers, in what is surely one of the most absurd jokes a playwright ever scripted for a player, *that he has been locked on the stage!*[17] Unexpectedly (did the play not seem over?), Firs begins the monologue which closes the comedy:

> [*goes up to the door and touches the handle*] Locked. They've gone away . . . [*Sits on the sofa.*] They forgot me . . . It's nothing . . . I'll sit here for a while . . . And Leonid Andreich didn't put on his fur coat, I suppose, he must have gone away in his light one . . .[*Sighs anxiously.*] I just didn't look after it . . . Oh, these green young things—they never learn! [*Mumbles something that cannot be understood.*] Life just slipped by as if I'd never even lived . . . [*Lies down.*] I'll lie down for a while . . . You just don't have any strength, none, nothing's left, nothing at all. . . . Oh, you . . . silly galoot, you! . . *He lies motionless. A sound is heard far off in the distance, as if coming from the sky. It is the sound of a string breaking that dies away sadly. A*

> *stillness falls, and nothing is heard but the sound of an axe striking a tree far away in the orchard.*
>
> [Pp. 210–11]

It is not easy to describe the effect in performance of the final moments of *The Cherry Orchard,* but it constitutes one of the most remarkably ironic closures in the history of the theater. For one thing, I can recall no other play which ends with an actor prone and motionless but not "dead." In the absolute cessation of visible histrionic effort we may glimpse a final image of the organizing *gest* of this comedy. It is appropriate that first silence and then offstage noises ironically counterpoint the actor's living but motionless presence. Styan notes that the final silence can be sustained for as long as a full minute and yet not lose its power, but the power is felt explicitly in terms of its ability to cause an audience to invest their selves in the play. They experience nothing less than the utter collapse of the play world. Here, as elsewhere, Chekhov compels his audience to reinvent a language that connects theater with world. Like many earlier comic playwrights, Chekhov focuses his drama on actors who take on roles, but now the playwright "celebrates" ironically the collapse of the protected world of comedy.[18]

It is impossible historically to separate Chekhov's dramaturgy from the naturalistic productions of the Moscow Art Theatre, though Chekhov's protests against Stanislavsky's methods and interpretations have become part of the lore of theater history. Yet in support of the reading which I have just proposed for *The Cherry Orchard,* I might add, finally, Meyerhold's observation that the Moscow Art Theatre, despite its early successes in performing Chekhov, very quickly lost the key to performing his drama. Too much emphasis on external elements—representational acting, infinitely detailed sets, sounds of crickets, and horses' hoofs—as Meyerhold has observed, soon obscured the fact that the entire success of performing Chekhov depended upon recognizing the actor as the most important element of the performance.[19] As for the exuberance with which Stanislavsky added sounds, we might observe in passing that *many* offstage noises very soon become accepted by an audience as part of the script, whereas a *few* random noises are perceived as a threat to the script and so create a vastly different response. The more frequent the sounds, the more they become anticipated and therefore regular in a phenomenological sense. Spectators may easily integrate them with the representational frame, so that they are not at all disconcerting or distracting—except, of course, to Chekhov's ears, which were listening for discord.

Furthermore, we might restate Meyerhold's meaning: the actor who plays, say, Ivan Voynitsky (*Uncle Vanya*) must know what it is like "realistically" to play a pitiable failure, but he must simultaneously attempt to play the stylized fool that Chekhov made the center of the third act's farce, and he must master *that* role and *that* situation by seeming visibly to fail in it, to fail, that is, at creating stock farce responses. Here, as was true of the actors in *The Cherry Orchard,* Chekhov's player attempts to make the familiar theatrical gestures, and yet those conventional responses seem no longer meaningful in ways which the audience anticipates. The result is comic theater with an interest in inventing new meaning for histrionic existence: what does it mean to miss a cue, to forget one's lines, to be unable to master one's emotions, to be given a farcical role which one can never live out? In the resulting crossover of motives—the actor who masters a farcical role partly by fumbling it—there arise the special characteristics of Chekhov's comic theater. It is a theater *about* comedy in the way that, say, Aristophanic comedy is a theater about contemporary Athenian tragedy; that is, in each instance the playwright creates meaning by innovative play with the givens of his age and its attitudes toward the theater.

Whatever the ultimate source of Chekhov's lifelong fascination with farce and vaudeville, his experimentation with those forms opened for himself and subsequent modern dramatists new ways to create comic theater. Chekhov discovered that it was possible for competent actors to play with familiar comic roles and to shape them into something quite unexpected. As earlier performance styles had circumscribed the meanings of comic theater within certain "horizons of expectation," so Chekhov's odd, dissonant dramaturgy allowed his actors to thrust those familiar roles out at the audience in aggressive new ways. In the last essay of this study, I shall examine a more recent comedy: Friedrich Dürrenmatt's *The Visit*. In his work we may see how contemporary comic playwrights continue to play with the received forms of comic theater in order to redefine them for individual ends.

6 Comedy, Community, and the Anonymous Audience: Dürrenmatt's *Der Besuch der alten Dame*

> And lastly it is through the conceit, through comedy that the anonymous audience becomes possible as an audience, becomes a reality to be counted on, and also, one to be taken into account. The conceit easily transforms the crowd of theatre-goers into a mass which can be attacked, deceived, outsmarted into listening to things it would otherwise not so readily listen to. Comedy is a mousetrap in which the public is easily caught and in which it will get caught over and over again. Tragedy, on the other hand, predicated a true community, a kind of community whose existence in our day is but an embarrassing fiction.
> —Friedrich Dürrenmatt, "Problems of the Theatre"

Whether the concept of genre enhances or retards appreciation of theater has always been a crucial question, if a vexing one. Everyone remembers that Socrates put his audience to sleep with a disquisition on tragedy and comedy, while more recent skeptics of genre theory have questioned *where* genres exist, if indeed they exist at all. Folk wisdom has it that the most successful dramatists ignore the critics' prescriptions; especially in the case of "absurdist" theater, playwrights and theorists seem unable to settle even the most basic issues.

The purpose of this final chapter is to make explicit an assumption that has shaped the discussion of comedy in this book: that even though there may be no "natural" genre of comedy, generic approaches to theater continue to be both relevant and useful. The mistake is to insist that there is a typical shape or end for comic theater, when the best available evidence suggests that in the periods when theater is most vital, comedy and tragedy are not stable dramatic forms but horizons of possibility which may be played off one against the other. One illustration may be found in the representation of death on stage. Generally speaking, until the twentieth century, comedies lacked corpses, whereas tragedies were of course littered with them. It was inevitable, then, to conclude that the appearance during the modern period of "comedies with corpses" signified an overall generic collapse.

But the situation is more problematic than it may first seem. For one thing, stage "deaths" are not phenomenologically distinct from other theatrical representations. What sense, then, does it make to argue that an audience interprets an actor's "death" as fundamentally different from any of his other actions? Othello is only "playing" at murdering Desdemona, as anyone (fools excepted) sitting in the audience can plainly "see"; her "death," therefore, may be "enjoyed" by an audience, just as may any of her other actions. The understanding especially for modern audiences is that spectators need not confront the Figur's plight because of its obvious confinement within the theatrical frame. This dying is not really addressed as dying but as a mode of "sport."

Rendering death as theater has obvious limits, as illustrated by the sometime Roman practice of fitting the executions of criminals into certain performances. The argument that they were going to be killed anyway always sounds bizarre. Or now, when death sentences are beginning again to be carried out in America, powerful restrictions operate to prevent executions from becoming "theater." States scrupulously permit only the minimum number of watchers necessary to establish the event as fact, as if more than three or four onlookers would make the drama of dying too much like drama—something done expressly for the visual consumption of an audience. The potential psychopathology of making the world into a stage is superbly illustrated by the anecdote of the anonymous German machine gunner who, hiding in his trench some two minutes before the Armistice ending World War I went into effect, suddenly fired from his weapon a continuous belt of ammunition. He then slowly rose, removed his helmet, and bowed grandly to the astonished British soldiers some hundred yards distant. He turned and, as if stepping through the folds of some invisible curtain, walked slowly away from his role in the Great War. By treating the theater of war literally as a theater, that soldier keyed his real life activity into the only possible framework which rendered it acceptable to him as human experience. War was indeed high comedy, his the starring role.[1]

The power of the modern theatrical frame conceptually to divorce actor from deed in this way is truly impressive. But the representational frame carries a corollary notion which for the purpose of understanding Dürrenmatt's comic theater is even more significant: that the watchers are obliged to refrain from participating in the actors' reality. They may look but never touch. No matter what they do, they cannot affect the actors; especially during a realistic production, the audience understands itself to be absent from the world being presented.

This freedom from actual involvement tends to be valued by many, but the privileged ontological status of modern watchers does not lack for critics. Nikolai Okholopov was experimenting during the 1930s with the physical mingling of actors and audiences in order to bring the two groups into closer emotional rapport, an ambition different in no fundamental way from the aims of Allan Kaprow, Jerzy Grotowski, or Richard Schechner. My contention is that some forms of modern comedy grow out of what may be termed a variety of the "antitheatrical prejudice."[2] Given "troubled times" and modern empathetic sensibilities, pleasure and laughter and even the theatrical frame can sometimes be seen as harmful excesses which need to be purged or possibly corrected. Making jokes is making theater, as both Freud and Bergson understood, and becoming an audience to another's acts is a way of making that person into a scapegoat. If we could devise, then, new modes of affective response which would eliminate schadenfreude from comedy, these ungenerous impulses would be checked. In *The Visit,* Dürrenmatt prescribes a remedy for spectators for whom playing the role of onlookers has become banal, depleted of humanity.

The events of *Der Besuch*[3] follow very closely the scapegoat myth. The action begins in a wasted, dying city: the men of Güllen, a fictional town situated somewhere in Europe, sit idle, while their community, suffering from economic depression, slowly withers. At first it seems that no one in particular is to blame for the town's poverty, but we are soon given evidence that the Gülleners' town has been mysteriously singled out for ruin. The whole surrounding countryside is booming, as it were; only Güllen goes bankrupt. The local villagers regard their suffering with increasing suspicion: its source is to be traced, or so they speculate, to the sinister conspiracies of Free Masons, Jews, Communists.

Dürrenmatt's donnée explicitly recalls one far older, in particular, the *Oedipus tyrannos* of Sophocles. It turns out that Güllen, like Thebes, is cursed because of an undisclosed crime committed by one of its citizens, now an eminent businessman and candidate for mayor. Forty-five years before the events dramatized in the play, a man named Alfred Ill falsely disclaimed responsibility for the child of a young girl, Clara Wäscher. Because he did not wish to marry Clara, Ill bribed two townsmen to testify in court that they, too, had slept with Clara. Publicly and wrongly shamed, Clara was forced to leave Güllen, and over the next decades, Ill married, fathered two children, and prospered, while Clara turned first to prostitution, then, miraculously, found good fortune and eventually became Claire Zachanassian, the richest lady in the world. The action of *The Visit* begins on the eve of Claire's homecoming. As the play begins, various townsfolk are decorating the village square. They picture a joyous reunion—not because they are particularly glad to see Claire, but because they hope that she will use some of her great wealth to relieve Güllen's plight.

When Claire arrives, however, the townsfolk learn that their recent series of misfortunes is not accidental. They discover that their woe results from Claire's revenge on the town that long ago cast her out. For a number of years she has systematically (but anonymously) purchased and dismantled all the local businesses and so has brought Güllen to the edge of absolute ruin. And her revenge has a final frightening twist: Claire offers a gift of one billion dollars to restore the town to economic health—but only in exchange for Ill's death.

The townspeople are shocked by her proposal, and at first they vigorously reject Claire's offer, loudly proclaiming their support for Ill. Indeed, at this point we are likely to be gratified by the Gülleners' moral integrity: it is simple, direct, genuine. The mayor expresses the villagers' outrage and moral integrity:

> Madam Zachanassian: We are still in Europe; we are still not savages. I reject your offer in the name of the city of Güllen. In the name of humanity. We would rather remain poor than blood-spattered.
>
> [P. 295]

To which Claire laconically replies: "I'll wait" (p. 295).

The Gülleners at this moment truly mean those words; they truly mean to do the moral thing. Ironically, however, the Gülleners' morals are strained to the breaking point not by the temptation of immense wealth and prosperity but by little, everyday pleasures. Claire continues to live among them; slowly, in her presence, the townspeople begin to buy cigarettes and milk and chocolate and shoes on credit, hoping that the crisis will vanish, that Claire will abandon the terrible condition of her largesse. She does not, and subtly the Gülleners' attitudes toward Ill and his old crime begin to change. The deeper their actual monetary debt, the more the Gülleners rationalize that "justice" must be obtained at any price. Ultimately they murder Ill, first ostracizing him and then strangling him with solemn formality. The play ends in a macabre celebration: having received Claire's check for a billion dollars, the Gülleners grow visibly more prosperous, until, richly clad in formal evening dress, men and women form two choruses to sing hymns to their newfound fortune:

Keep the night at bay,
Nevermore let it darken our city
Risen anew, magnificent.

[P. 356]

What meaning may be derived from this sequence of events? For many readers, the answer lies in Dürrenmatt's updated telling of a tale which has been told countless times before. Even when it was new to the stage, *The Visit* seemed in many ways an ancient work, one which offered its spectators access to the archaic, ritual roots of tragic theater. Some years ago, for example, Melvin Askew wrote:

> The power of *Der Besuch,* like the power of *Oedipus Rex* or *Oedipus at Colonnus,* derives in great part from its reduction of life to ritual, but the most astonishing and the most profound effect of the play derives—unlike the effect of *Oedipus Rex*— almost exclusively from its successful ritualization and confirmation of some of the deepest, blackest, and perhaps most intolerable suspicions of modern man, as well as by its presentation of an almost hopelessly complex and ambiguous moral issue, one, in fact, which makes those same qualities in Hawthorne and Melville seem almost innocent and secure. The central figure by which this artistic compression and ideological and emotional ritualization occurs is, of course, Madame Zachanassian and especially by her association with the Sphinx.[4]

Dürrenmatt orients his play specifically toward Greek tragedy, and in doing so he pursues a literary method common to many modern writers: that is, he orders scenes from contemporary life by playing them against a mythic background. These facts about the structure of *The Visit* have long been apparent; anyone who reads or sees Dürrenmatt's play cannot help but notice the conscious effort the playwright makes to link his drama with ancient tragic theater. I am interested here in exploring an aspect of *The Visit* which has so far received little attention but will illustrate how Dürrenmatt creates theater by using comedy to create an audience.

When the action of *The Visit* begins, a number of the citizens of Güllen have assembled at the train station, waiting:

> THE FIRST. The *Gudrun,* Hamburg-Naples.
> THE SECOND. At eleven twenty-seven the *Racing Roland* arrives, Venice-Stockholm.
> THE THIRD. The only pleasure we have left: watching trains.
> THE FOURTH. Five years ago the *Gudrun* and the *Racing Roland* stopped in Güllen. Also the *Diplomat* and the *Lorelei,* all famous express trains.
> THE FIRST. World famous.
> THE SECOND. Now even the commuter trains don't stop. Only two from Kaffigen and the one-thirteen from Kalberstadt.
> THE THIRD. Ruined.
> THE FOURTH. The Wagner factory collapsed.
> THE FIRST. Bockmann bankrupt.
> THE SECOND. The foundry on Sunshine Square gone under.
> THE THIRD. Life on unemployment compensation.
> THE FOURTH. In soup lines.
> THE FIRST. Life?
> THE SECOND. Vegetating.
> THE THIRD. Rotting.
> THE FOURTH. The whole town.
> *Bell tolls*
>
> [Pp. 269–70]

Such language typifies the speech patterns of the Gülleners just before the arrival of Claire Zachanassian, and its effect in these opening moments of the performance is galvanic. The dialogue, though sparse, is skillfully packed with expository information. The men's conversation is not wooden but intensely dramatic, and from their present situation springs their hopes for the town's future:

> THE SECOND. High time the millionairess came. In Kalberstadt they say she financed a hospital.
>
> [P. 270]

I have followed Dürrenmatt's German as closely as possible in English, both in vocabulary and in syntax, so as to be able to make several points regarding the histrionic effects of Dürrenmatt's dialogue. The most noticeable characteristic of his language is its ability to establish, despite its extreme terseness, a very strong sense of forward movement. Each speech, however short, however it may appear visibly to repeat the one before it, fairly bristles with possibilities and causes onlookers to anticipate new statements, new questions, new directions. Momentum subtly builds throughout the first several speeches; it increases steadily through the linguistic sequence "watching trains" and "all famous express trains," until it reaches a peak with the First Man's intensifier, "world famous." Then, with the following remark, the men's commentary on the past thrusts forward into the present: *"Now* [italics mine] even the commuter trains don't stop" (*Nun halten nicht einmal die Personenzüge*). Afterward a new linguistic structure is introduced—a play, almost musical in its effect upon an audience, of inflected verbals: "ruined," "collapsed," "gone under" (*ruiniert, zusammengekracht, eingegangen*). And the counterpoint to this rhythm occurs in the patterns of verbal response to the First Man's rhetorical query, "Life?"—"vegetating," "rotting," "the whole town" (*vegetieren, krepieren, Das ganze Städtchen*). The language here brilliantly illustrates Susanne Langer's meaning when she compared the language of a play to a runner in motion, whose speed depends upon his using the energy of one stride to carry him forward to the next.[5] Dürrenmatt's dialogue is intensely *dramatic*.

Of this language, Askew writes: "Here is the language of ritual, spoken by the faceless and representative characters, the devotee or the priest, and here too is language as highly stylized and as ritualistic as the stychomythia of Greek tragedy."[6] This is a puzzling way to describe the introductory scene of *The Visit,* and to call such language "ritualistic" is highly inaccurate—though, to be sure, Askew's use of the term is characteristic of the very imprecise (and very misleading) way this concept has for many years figured in the criticism of drama.[7] Simply put, a ritual action is one which manifests for spectators certain consciously shared formulas. Thus, in order to imagine that these men's words and actions enact "ritual" theater, we must imagine first of all that they have lived this scene innumerable times before and, second, that their language constitutes *in cooperation with the audience* a shared system of belief. To believe the former makes nonsense of some of the men's remarks, and to believe the second is frankly impossible.

Moreover, ritual language is specifically *atemporal*. The rite—any rite—obliterates or transcends time, therefore any truly ritual language contains powerful checks against temporality.[8] In contrast, the introductory scene of *The Visit* stresses time's passing: trains go by, keeping time to the minute; factories crash, foundries shut down, townships rot, hospitals are built, fortunes made, heritages lost, inns visited, and music—sound patterns in time—is composed. The scene begins and ends with the tolling of a bell. And this wealth of temporal change is further enriched by the strong impression of linear progress which inheres in Dürrenmatt's syntax. From every perspective, the basis of this introductory scene appears to be time and change; how, then, can one possibly call this action *ritualized*? Highly *stylized*, to be sure; but the overall impression is not of life reduced to ritual but of life historicized. The action in the town possesses a unique pace, beat, feel. *The Visit* begins *in* time and proceeds, during the introductory moments, *on* time—for all goes according to schedule until Claire Zachanassian arrives.

Contrast the language of the Gülleners (the *visited*) with the language that arrives along with the *visitors*. Claire's arrival itself is anachronous: she comes neither on the right train nor at the right time. Soon afterward, the audience meets a mysterious pair of *castrati*. Their entrance comes almost as an afterthought. Just as the stage empties of Gülleners and maidservants and an almost endless stream of cases and trunks, there stroll into view, in Dürrenmatt's description, "two short, fat, old men with soft voices, hands held out, very carefully dressed" (p. 282). And with the pair comes a sudden change in the mood of the play. They are blind, and their commentary arouses the curiosity of a nearby policeman:

> THE PAIR. We are in Güllen. We smell it, we smell it, we smell it in the air, in the Güllen air.
> POLICEMAN. Who are you then?
> THE PAIR. We belong to the old lady, we belong to the old lady. She calls us Koby and Loby.
> POLICEMAN. Madame Zachanassian is staying at the Golden Apostle.
> THE PAIR. (*gaily*) We are blind, we are blind.
> POLICEMAN. Blind? Then I'll take you there, two times.

THE PAIR. Thanks, Mister Policeman, thanks very much.
POLICEMAN. (*surprised*) How did you know that I was a policeman, if you are blind?
THE PAIR. By your tone, by your tone, all policemen have the same tone.

[P. 282]

It is worthwhile to consider what response this scene evokes from an audience. So far, the tone of the play has not been particularly sinister; in fact, once Claire arrives, the play takes on the appearance of a ludicrous spectacle, one dominated by a ridiculous old lady dressed in unbelievably grotesque fashion: red hair, bangles, pearl necklace, the works. And to the extent that the audience is pleased to witness all the bustle associated with Claire's arrival, it feels initially the impulse to treat the blind pair as one more ludicrous component of Claire's ludicrous retinue—objects, that is, whose chief purpose is to provide them with an amusing piece of theater. When the visitors appear, however, they introduce speech rhythms which clash absurdly with the normal rhythms of the "visited." The castrati, Koby and Loby, bring with them pathological language, a language which, like them, has been unsexed. Their speech is equivocal, split by meaningless antitheses. As the policeman comments, "These foreigners have a funny humor" (p. 283).

Two words from his observation are especially significant: "funny" (*komischen*) and "foreigners" (*Ausländer*). The policeman's comment is more a defense mechanism than a rational analysis, and at this point his remarks probably reflect the opinions of Dürrenmatt's audience. Audiences have always liked to see people very different from themselves on stage. Often, of course, they call such creatures "funny."

Curiously, this pair does not seem particularly laughable, yet it ought to be supremely funny. Twins have long been stock figures of fun in the theater, and mindlessly repetitive characters such as these almost always evoke laughter on the part of the beholder. Comic playwrights have always known that unincremental repetition is funny, and characters who are unknowingly mired in their own language have long been stock figures of fun in the theater. Henri Bergson found in such thoughtless behavior evidence that something mechanical had become "encrusted" on something living, that the élan vital, whose essence was flux, was behaving like a factory machine. People behave this way, Bergson theorized, whenever they do not pay sufficient attention to their situation. This absentmindedness, he said, was detrimental to the continuing health of society, and so, to correct this threat to its well-being, society laughs.[9]

Bergson says in "Laughter," "We laugh every time a person gives us the impression of being a thing,"[10] and, in fact, *The Visit* could profitably be interpreted as an elaborate disquisition on his essay. Koby and Loby are not the only people in the comedy who have been made into objects. Claire's appearance is grotesque, obviously made up; moreover, as she displays at least two artificial limbs, she is already part "thing." Too, the obvious doublings of characters (Koby/Loby, Roby/Toby) connote a comic assembly line. Husbands can apparently be factory produced: Claire arrives with husband-to-be number eight, whom she marries in Güllen and promptly divorces before proceeding to number nine. And the Gülleners, insofar as their experience over the course of the play's action can be summarized, begin as people and end as robots.

Yet anyone who reads Dürrenmatt's postscript, as well as his theoretical essay "Problems of the Theatre," knows that the author does not intend his drama to be played exclusively for laughs. Dürrenmatt especially condemns audiences who accept comedy "only when it makes people feel as bestially happy as a bunch of pigs."[11] In the particular case of *The Visit,* the playwright enjoins a stock humorous response. He terms Claire and the two eunuchs, Koby and Loby, "poetical apparitions." "The Eunuchs," he specifies, "are not to be given a realistic, unappetizing interpretation, with gelded voices, but must seem improbable, like a fairy tale, soft, ghostly in their plant-like existence, a sacrifice to total revenge, whose logic is the law books of antiquity" (p. 358).

Dürrenmatt demands much of the actors who play this pair, insisting that they achieve a complex performance style within the limits of two brief scenes, and it will be illustrative to consider these otherwise minor characters in some detail. In order to achieve the effect that Dürrenmatt's production notes indicate, the actors who play Koby and Loby must unsettle their spectators by approaching the roles of comic butts in a new and provocative manner. Dürrenmatt does *not* want his actors to "humanize" their clowns' masks, nor does he count to any great extent on spectators' sympathizing with them because of their cruel treatment at the hands of Claire Zachanassian. It is clear that the problem for the actors who play Koby and Loby is to keep their performance from either of two recognizable extremes. They must avoid spilling over into sentimentalism, on the one hand, or farce, on the other, and the best way for them to do so is for the actors to pretend that they have been estranged from their roles as buffoons.

We may imagine Koby and Loby dressed alike, stock buffoons ostensibly ready to perform their mechanized comic routines for the delight of the onlookers. Yet the anticipated comedic performance never materializes. For a spectator the performance of Koby and Loby proves unusually disquieting because it is so obviously at odds with the farcical text which seems to have been written for them. It is always upsetting to discover sudden changes in familiar behavioral patterns, whether in real life or onstage; in the case of Koby and Loby, however, an audience is not really asked to deal with changes in ostensibly human behavior. Because Koby and Loby are conceived not as people but as mechanisms, the response of the audience instead derives from a renewed perspective on "comic" mechanical behavior. Onlookers are prepared to respond to the castrati as children to their wind-up toys, and the confused annoyance that an audience feels when confronted with Koby and Loby resembles that of a small child whose mechanical robot, which had been performing with great zest, suddenly and mysteriously runs down. Koby and Loby must appear to be "dead" theatrically. They seem like two clowns whose mainspring has been broken, and their performance as a consequence takes on the dimensions of something uncanny. Herein lies the brilliant inventiveness of the echolalia which Dürrenmatt creates for them to speak. It *ought* to be supremely funny, but its retarded tempo only underscores the weird disjunction between "comic" text and estranged performance.[12]

Spectators' inevitable error in framing the performance of Koby and Loby typifies the overall method by which Dürrenmatt transforms his audience from comedic anonymity to full communal responsibility, implicating them ultimately in Ill's death for their willingness to be spectators only. This process of emotional involvement takes place gradually. Partway through Act 2, for example, Dürrenmatt dramatizes a scene which presents the first evidence of the changes being wrought in Güllen. Two women enter Ill's store, intending to purchase some milk:

FIRST WOMAN: Milk, Mr.Ill.
SECOND WOMAN: My can, Mr. Ill.
ILL: A hearty good morning. A liter of milk for the ladies.
(He opens a milkcan and starts to dip milk.)
FIRST WOMAN: Whole milk, Mr. Ill.
SECOND WOMAN: Two liters of whole milk, Mr. Ill.
ILL: Whole milk.
(He opens another can and dips milk.)

[P. 299]

Later, in the same act, a similar scene occurs:

THE FIRST: We'll stand by you. By *our* Ill. Rock-steady.
THE WOMEN: *Eating chocolate:* Rock-steady, Mr. Ill, rock-steady.
THE SECOND: You are certainly our most beloved personality.
THE FIRST: The most important.
THE SECOND: You'll be elected mayor in spring.
THE FIRST: Dead certain.
THE WOMEN: *Eating chocolate:* Dead certain, Mr. Ill, dead certain.

[P. 301]

The Gülleners' metamorphosis is not complete at this stage, for elsewhere in this scene the women converse normally, as do a number of other customers. It is part of Dürrenmatt's design to dramatize gradual, and not sudden, change. These events are not to be understood as anything the town's inhabitants are conscious of, and it is certainly not something they intend; indeed, as Dürrenmatt specifies, the Gülleners who slaughter Ill are "people like all of us," and "they are certainly not to be portrayed as wicked." "At first," Dürrenmatt writes, "they are decided to reject the offer; to be sure, they incur debts, but that is not because of their intention to kill Ill, but out of thoughtlessness, out of a feeling that everything will work itself out happily. The Second Act should be directed accordingly" (p. 359).

The change which Dürrenmatt summarizes is manifest largely as a transition from one performance mode to another. The most visible evidence of this transition is the gradual substitution of echolalia for the dramatically conventional language which the four men use in Act I as they sit watching the trains go by. It is ironic that this change is finally accomplished back at the train station, when, at the end of Act II, Ill attempts to leave a town whose citizens now behave in a menacing way. Here, finally, the Gülleners first display group behavior:

> THE MAYOR: That is your train.
> ALL: Your train! Your train!
> THE MAYOR: Now, Ill, I wish you a good trip.
> ALL: A good trip, a good trip!
> THE DOCTOR: A happy, long life.
> ALL: A happy, long life.
> *(The Gülleners crowd around Ill.)*
> THE MAYOR: It's time to get on. Climb on the commuter train to Kalberstadt; go in God's name.
> THE POLICEMAN: And good luck in Australia!
> ALL: Good luck, good luck!
>
> [P. 317]

By now the audience is fully conscious of Ill's peril. The spectators know that he is trapped, and this knowledge renders the events of the final act—the formal expulsion, the strangling, the concluding hymn—terrible but necessary. This mindless group behavior is appalling to behold, but *The Visit* does not achieve its impressive histrionic force because it "imitates" ritual behavior nor even because it depicts the substitution of mindless sacrificial rite for acts of will. Rather, as was true of *The Cherry Orchard, The Visit* depends for its histrionic force on actors who weirdly redefine the theatrical frame an audience expects to apply during the performance of drama. It is vital to the success of this play that onlookers first experience the "normal" energies of drama in the introductory scene, for only then can they feel threatened by the contrasting "funny" modes of behavior which arrive with the foreigners.

Clearly, Dürrenmatt wants his spectators to anticipate a performance rhythm of one sort, so that he can challenge them by supplying a different one. The interplay between these two performance styles, one conventionally dramatic and moving *in* time, and one abnormal, moving *out* of time, constitutes the working power of *The Visit*.

This transformation constitutes not simply the "ritualization" of life in Güllen but rather its immoral *theatricalization*.[13] Claire desires revenge, but her revenge takes a peculiar form: she wants the world made into a spectacle for her own private amusement. In her imagination, the world is a stage, a stage peopled with fools, and—unfortunately—she has the power to impose her imaginative fictions on the world. That the world (here represented by Güllen) contains nothing but fools is a view that, as Stanley Cavell has observed, necessarily implicates its proponent.[14] At bottom, Claire's proposal is most repugnant not because she wants "justice" or even revenge but because she dehumanizes people by turning them into players for her own objective contemplation. *The Visit*, in this respect, is less concerned to imitate the scapegoat ritual than to implicate spectators in the psychology by which scapegoats are created. And the way to create scapegoats in the easiest manner and with the least attendant guilt is to put them on a stage where they may be contemplated safely by a group. If the stage has a proscenium arch, and if the seating area is darkened, so much the better.

Once Claire arrives in town, she establishes residence at the Golden Apostle and begins to contemplate the folly of the townsfolk from the detached, audiencelike vantage point of her balcony. Insofar as spectators share her *perspective* (it is not necessary to sympathize with her ambitions for Ill's murder), they implicate themselves in her monstrosity. The mise-en-scène of Act II stresses such a theatricalization of Güllen, as the stage here is separated into several playing areas: in the foreground, stage left and stage right, respectively, are the police station and Ill's store, while in the background is the exterior of the hotel Golden Apostle. Claire is seated on her balcony, raised above the main playing level, so as to give the impression that she is a spectator to events in town. Her position mirrors that of an audience, monitor to an ongoing series of events. At this stage, however, the play's spectators do not realize the immorality of Claire's activity because they are busily engaged in doing what she is doing: watching, watching passively, unobserved and unacknowledged by the players. In failing to understand what Claire's true activity is, the onlookers fail to see their own error: that they too are keeping themselves aloof from the "characters" who exist exclusively for their objective contemplation.

By passively accepting the theatrical frame, the spectators understand that they are to remain mute witnesses to the actions on stage. Dürrenmatt means *The Visit* to overcome this essentially disengaged role of onlooker. We might express his point thus: the trouble with going to the theater is that we are sometimes tempted to believe that nothing onstage is really happening—that the actors are just playing games, that the people visible are just "characters" whose exclusively fictional status releases viewers from the need to engage the actor/characters in their problematic humanity. But this is playing the role of the spectator with a vengeance: hidden in the dark, accountable to nothing and to no one, we grow to resemble Claire Zachanassian, refusing to acknowledge *these people,* refusing to admit the claims that their lives make. It is no accident that Claire plans to take Ill's body back with her: he will lie forever, she muses, in a mausoleum in Capri, where only she can see him. This grotesque tableau constitutes the logical end of Claire's passion for making the world her stage. It is the ultimate gest of *The Visit.* As Claire epitomizes the spectator, so Ill, in turn, becomes the epitome of the actor who dares not address the unseen spectators. Eternally frozen in his death mask, eternally pleasing to his silent audience, Ill makes no claims whatsoever on the onlooker. His only purpose is to please. We could go so far as to say that *The Visit* constitutes an ironic commentary on the representational frame—ideally, the living actors are obliged to "play dead" behind their masks.

In this respect, the only essential difference between Claire and Dürrenmatt's audience is that she is *on*stage, and so is physically in a position to acknowledge Ill, while spectators offstage are not.

Her amusement derives from her own willed detachment from the situation, from the fact that she literally does nothing to accomplish her desires: she does not have to participate in Ill's slaughter. She merely watches. The pain of Dürrenmatt's audience, on the other hand, derives from the belated acknowledgment that, while they *would* intervene in events if they could, they are powerless to do so. They do not intervene, of course, because such are the conventions of representational theater: faced with the most grisly murder, spectators are powerless, they do nothing. They cannot even cry out, as the children do for Tinkerbell. *The Visit* not only dramatizes this theme but also compels audiences to experience it. Central to the experience of this play is the discovery that we must suffer for the failure to speak out, for dissociating ourselves from the world. The onlookers' experience is deepened, made more painful and perhaps more meaningful, because they are first invited to take the position from which the staged events seem comic spectacle: "From the right comes Claire Zachanassian, sixty-two, red hair, pearl necklace, giant gold bangles, 'dressed to kill,' impossible" (p. 275). Eventually it occurs to an audience that Claire is not just one more ludicrous buffoon but is literally "dressed to kill" (*aufgedonnert*). But the spectators learn simultaneously that they cannot alter their role as onlookers. They are thus made victims of their own lust for spectacle as surely as Ill is vicitimzed by Claire.

The point of *The Visit,* then, is intentionally and explicitly theatrical, intentionally and explicitly moralistic: it is immoral to address the world as a spectator. In "Problems of the Theatre," Dürrenmatt wrote, "The world is far bigger than any man, and perforce threatens him constantly. If one could but stand outside the world, it would no longer be threatening. But I have neither the right nor the ability to be an outsider to this world. To find solace in poetry can also be all too cheap; it is more honest to retain one's human point of view."[15] If only we could stay in the audience! But that detached position, as Dürrenmatt sees it, is "comic"; to assume it is to play audience to other's acts, to put oneself in Claire's place. It is no accident that Claire is the only character in *The Visit* with a sense of humor; indeed, the many speeches in which she wryly assesses her previous husbands are engagingly funny. But we cannot, given the terms of this comedy, play the amused spectator, making other human beings the objects of our own dispassionate interest. How is it possible to claim the privileges of a spectator without abandoning our humanity? How is it possible to make someone the object of a group's interest without denying that person's humanness? And how is it possible to remain hidden from others without becoming, like Claire, a monster? without saying, in effect, *these people do not matter to me?*

In any case, *The Visit* is remarkable not only for its ritual content or its political ideology but also for its curious antitheatrical bias. Here the *rejection* of theater serves as a standard of moral worth. There is hope manifest in this play, not onstage but offstage. Here the search for authenticity requires that the spectators play their roles in order to deny them. Dürrenmatt requires his audience to live through the dilemma of being mute observers. Their freedom is not that they are in the audience, but that, suffering through the experience of being watchers, they can reject the onlookers' role of separateness. By reminding audiences of their continuing human commitments, *The Visit* obligates them to examine the consequences of their desires for spectacle. The initial lust for spectacle transforms them eventually into wiser participants. They survive the play so that, leaving the playhouse, they may reaffirm their commitment to community and to each other. And in this inverted fashion, the "comedy" of *The Visit* returns an audience to the communal experience of classical tragedy.

Afterword: On Actors and Theatrical Genres

> Comedy is an art form that arises naturally wherever people are gathered to celebrate life, in spring festivals, triumphs, birthdays, weddings, or initiations.
> —Susanne Langer, *Feeling and Form*

> We must beware of accepting obvious truths as more basic than others less obvious which are equally true and no less basic.
> —James K. Feibleman, *In Praise of Comedy*

I have offered in this book only a small number of specific readings of comedies. My aim has been to seek the meaning of a genre according to its perceptual basis, as a mode of histrionic performance. Rather than promulgate an entirely new theory of comedy, I have tried to suggest some alternate perspectives for understanding a few of the dimensions of comic performance and of theater generally, whether for the individual spectator or for the community. Anyone who has ever sat in a theater knows that the stage is not a source of prerecorded information and that spectators are not passive cryptologists. If anything, the onlookers not only complete the theater event but are themselves a source of meaning.

Some tentative conclusions, then. Drama, says Meyerhold, is the art of the actor. To behave like an actor is to find authenticity by behaving inauthentically. Inventing a self from nothing constitutes a mode of behavior so alien that it is probably impossible for the watchers ever to feel entirely comfortable with it. There is always something incalculably unstable about what actors do: never a guarantee, never a certainty that the circuit they hazard can be negotiated without peril. Whether we opt for "role making" or for "role taking," the results are the same. To be fashioned by Others is to lose ourselves in a script we did not write, but to opt to create the role we must first lay down what is most truly our own. In this process, inevitably, something cannot be grasped; something about living in the theater falsifies, equivocates, dissolves. "We cannot act what cannot be thought," says Herbert Blau, "and there's the promise. But even as the assertion is made, there is something in the theater which says: don't count on it."[1]

It is a difficult point to concede. The actor extends to spectators the promise of appearances, and his ventures enact their own problematic struggles to be: *that* self-image, *that* ideal person, not this one. (The appeal of the theater, Nicolas Evreinoff once remarked, is "the desire to be 'different,' to do something that is 'different,' to imagine oneself in surroundings that are 'different' from the commonplace surroundings of our everyday life.")[2] This compulsion to be different sometimes seems an unambiguous motive, as if the actors' metamorphic potential were uniformly attractive to audiences. But plays belie this statement: Mnesilochus enchained, Epidicus threatened with flogging, Overdo in the stocks, Argan tormented, Ill in his death mask. Theater is indeed transformation, but if spectators find pleasure in watching the actors' metamorphoses, they find pleasure too in making them hold still.

Making the actors hold still: in one guise or another, this is invariably part of spectators' pleasure in the theater. We sometimes imagine that drama differs in no essential way from any other literary art, that the play, like the narrative or even the lyric poem, is just one more way of telling a story. But of course it is not, and the confrontation of actors and watchers addresses desires and needs radically different from those which attend the narrative event. "The pivotal mechanism," writes Blau, "is the idea of punishment. . . . In the great ages of theater, punishment was up front, and bewildering. In our own period, it may be alternately up front or subliminal, strategically distributed or a function of new modalities of power, mass slaughter or minor cruelties, insidiously lenient, but still bewildering. As for the use of punishment, that still remains to be seen."[3] Theater is indeed imitation; but dramatic imitation is unlike that of the plastic or literary arts. The rhythm of imitation in the theater is aggressive, hostile, sometimes even fearful. There is no acting without violence, nor watching without identification, nor drama without some mode of punishment for the actor/character who takes on the blasphemous freedoms characteristic of his age.[4] And the varying dialectics which develop from the confrontation of performer and beholder are the wellsprings of power and meaning in the theater.

We might hope to conclude a book on comic theater on a less depressing note. Trying, therefore, to be as cheerful as possible (as Kenneth Burke once counseled when faced with evidence that humans tend to form groups by means of sacrificial pressures), we might distinguish between virtual and actual victimage. "Victimage," Burke says, "is *not inevitable*";[5] only its temptation is. In this case comic theater is neither exclusively celebratory nor fundamentally stabilizing. Indeed, it is a mode of theater considerably more radical than tragedy because it partly denies audiences the sacrificial motives they come to the theater seeking to pursue.

The evidence provided by the plays that I have discussed suggests that the actor is more visible in comedy than in tragedy. Now and then this extra dimension of the comedic performance is said to reflect comic theater's essentially nonserious nature: its emphasis on "play" or on "game" or its status as a consciously "socializing" institution. Without denying these truths, I would prefer also to describe the six comedies of this study as fundamentally learning theater. Each signifies a process that develops in the onlookers the ability to concentrate their entire psychic life (whatever their ambivalent feelings toward persona or player) into a coherent structure of growth and development. Tragedy conserves social value by exclusion, but these comedies, insofar as each insists upon the role of the player and the approach to the performance, subvert by combining identification with practical differentiation. The actor imprints on audiences not only an "identity" but also the theme of "identifying with"—a process which, while it does not rule out a compensatory exorcism or scapegoating, at least affords spectators greater opportunity to integrate or to "pool" the various objects, identifications, and frames of reference upon which individual and social development are founded.

Of course this is a "socializing" process, but "socializing" here refers to an activity considerably more problematic than is commonly granted to comedy. For one thing, the process is by no means without risks, nor is its end clearly foreseeable. The theater traditionally is a volatile place, and it is not always possible to predict the ends to which histrionic performance can lead a group of onlookers. As Brecht some years ago observed, we sometimes forget that human education proceeds along theatrical lines; if behavior arises from emotion, which cannot be taught, it is equally true that emotion arises from behavior, which can. We cannot, in other words, shrug off the political and moral implications of theater—in Brecht's words, "good when it is good, bad when it is bad."[6]

Fruitful discussion of theater presupposes more than aesthetic definitions of such terms as "character," "identification," and "imitation," among others. Admittedly these terms continue to tie criticism of drama to the familiar vocabulary of Aristotle, but we can at least use these words with greater appreciation of their fundamental mystery. "Identification," for example, as that term is loosely used in criticism of drama, masks a complex series of critical psychic operations; it is by means of a series of identifications that the personality is created. If the theater leads to fundamental "identifications," as it doubtless sometimes can, then aesthetics suddenly becomes ethics. Merely to admit the possibility of its doing so underscores Brecht's objections to empathy and opens new perspectives on two and a half millennia of antitheatrical polemic. I am not suggesting that literary scholars reenter the ancient debate between the theater and its critics. I mean that, if scholars see plays truly, theater offers renewed possibilities for understanding the relationship between the life of a society and the strategies of its art. Comedy in this broad sense describes both plays and their audiences. Past and present comedies, then, are neither the only right ones nor the only possible manifestations of comic theater.

Notes

Introduction

1. William Chetwood, *A General History of the Stage* (London, 1749); cited in Katharine Eisaman Maus, "'Playhouse Flesh and Blood,'" p. 599.
2. Henri Bergson, "Laughter," in *Comedy*, introd. Wylie Sypher, p. 123.
3. Maus, "'Playhouse Flesh and Blood,'" p. 601.
4. *Lysistrata*, trans. B. B. Rogers, p. 107, n. *d*. Rogers omits part of this scene.
5. *Binetiomen;* my translation.
6. The descriptions of Macklin's performance are from *The Dramatic Censor*, quoted in A. M. Nagler, *A Source Book in Theatrical History*, p. 358.
7. These accounts of Kean's performance may be found in the Arden edition of *The Merchant of Venice*, ed. John Russell Brown, pp. xxxiii–xxxiv. Much of my summary of the transformations of Shylock's role is taken from the introduction to the comedy in the Arden edition, especially the "Stage History," pp. xxxii–xxxvi.
8. J. L. Styan, "Changeable Taffeta," p. 136.
9. Kenneth Burke, *The Philosophy of Literary Form*, pp. 70, 71.
10. The terms appear frequently in Brecht's theater criticism and are useful although they remain incompletely defined. See Patrice Pavis, *Languages of the Stage*, pp. 37–49: "On Brecht's Notion of *Gestus*." Many of Brecht's writings on theater are collected in *Brecht on Theatre*; see esp. pp. 104–6, 115–20, and 198–201.
11. See Pavis, *Languages of the Stage:* "It [*Gestus*] is a tool which remains exterior to the text, just as a seismograph is capable of recording the shakings of the earth without being a part of that shaking" (p. 48).
12. "Histrionic force" and its definition are borrowed from Michael Goldman, *The Actor's Freedom*, p. 77.
13. See Jean E. Howard, "Figures and Grounds": "It is a mistake . . . to assume that criticism concerned with a play's designs upon the audience must limit itself to a record of responses to a single actual pro-

duction. . . . I suggest, then, that critics concerned with understanding the strategies by which a playwright controls the responses of the audience must begin with the playscript itself, not with any one enactment of it" (p. 186).

14. My debt to Goffman is large. The few terms I mention here are inadequate to suggest the extent to which this study leans on his ideas. I cite relevant passages of *Frame Analysis* as they occur in the context of my discussions of individual comedies.

15. Goldman uses the term "actor-as-character," p. 6 and passim. Occasionally I distinguish between the "actor-character" and the persona: Dicaeopolis the alloy of player and role and Dicaeopolis the fiction.

1. Dramatic Illusion in Greek Old Comedy

1. My text is the Loeb Classical Library edition of Aristophanes, trans. B. B. Rogers; unless otherwise noted, all quotations follow Rogers's translations.

2. See Francisco R. Adrados, *Festival, Comedy, and Tragedy*, pp. 37–44.

3. I follow here Alastair Fowler's theory of genre, in *Kinds of Literature*, pp. 20–36.

4. See Francis Macdonald Cornford, *The Origin of Attic Comedy*, esp. chap. 4 ("Some Types of Dramatic Fertility Ritual") and chap. 9 ("Comedy and Tragedy").

5. See Sir Arthur Pickard-Cambridge, *Dithyramb, Tragedy, and Comedy*, pp. 192–94. Despite frequent criticism, Cornford's theory has proved central to discussions of comedy. At the center of Wylie Sypher's seminal essay on comedy we find Cornford's notion: comedy is "the ancient rite that is a Debate and a Carnival, a Sacrifice and a Feast." This synthesis of rational and irrational motives has proved compellingly attractive to comic theorists; as Morton Gurewitch concludes, "In actuality, the temptation to consider Cornford's views a godsend remains strong among theorists of comedy." The quoted statements appear in Sypher, *Comedy*, p. 255, and in Gurewitch, *Comedy: The Irrational Vision*, p. 41.

6. See Froma I. Zeitlin, "Cultic Models of the Female," pp. 129–33.

7. See Roger Caillois, *Man, Play, and Games;* Jacques Ehrmann, "Homo Ludens Revisited"; Johan Huizinga, *Homo Ludens;* Helen B. Schwartzman, *Transformations;* Phillips Stevens, Jr., ed., *Studies in the Anthropology of Play*, esp. pp. 250–65, a bibliography of play studies; Victor Turner, *The Ritual Process* and *Dramas, Fields, and Metaphors;* and

Roy Wagner, *Habu*. Wagner urges us to reorient our presuppositions with respect to the forms which societies "inherit" or "borrow" from their forbears: "The simple premise of innovation, that culture exists only through growth and transformation, underlies much of what seems basic in human activity, from the 'incest taboo' to the forms through which meaning is created. Technology is only a special case of this, as are naming, artistic creativity, and the practices that we call 'religious.' Whether we 'borrow' power and meaning from nature itself, from the forms and designations of our own culture or from those of exotic cultures, the significant factor is the mode of borrowing and transformation, not the content of that which is borrowed. The ethnographic content of a culture is thus merely a result, a cumulative historical increment of its transformations and a continuing 'context' for the formation of new metaphors. The life of the culture, its creations, revelations, activities, and strategies, is carried on through innovational styles" (p. 173).

8. See David Bain, *Actors and Audience*, p. 94.

9. See Peter Rau, *Paratragodia*. Rau argues that Aristophanes, in creating his comedies, plays freely with tragedy and so moves beyond tragedy to realize an ideal comic dramatic form: "Aristophanes's paratragedy is also characterized through that which is above all the animating principle of his comedy: through the *free play* with form, content, and application. In this free play between trivial reality, foolish farce, and the pathetic tragic ideal lies the real poetic basis of Aristophanic paratragedy" (pp. 183–84; my translation).

10. Bain, *Actors and Audience*, p. 96.

11. See Froma I. Zeitlin, "Travesties of Gender and Genre," p. 177.

12. Thus Cedric Whitman, in *Aristophanes and the Comic Hero*, writes, "*Thesmophoriazusae*, though one of the cleverest and funniest of the plays, at no point reflects any strong, general human feeling; it appeals to no widely acknowledged or intuited concern of either individual or society at large" (p. 217). Nevertheless, Whitman's study is still the best overall interpretation of Aristophanic comedy to date; any criticism of Old Comedy starts from his readings of the plays.

13. Zeitlin, "Travesties of Gender and Genre," pp. 170–71. I discovered Zeitlin's provocative and informative essay on *Thesmophoriazusae* only after much of my own work on the play had been completed. Her reading of Aristophanes' comedy occasionally anticipates mine but usually runs parallel to it. When appropriate, I cite her essay for support or clarification. See also my general essay on Aristophanic comedy, "Systematized Delirium."

14. On the polarization of theatrical genres in ancient Greece, see Adrados, *Festival, Comedy, and Tragedy*, also William E. Gruber, "The Polarization of Tragedy and Comedy." On the psychic life of fifth-century

Athenians, see Pedro Laín Entralgo, *The Therapy of the Word in Classical Antiquity;* citing E. Rohde's *Psyche,* Laín Entralgo writes: "the epidemic spread of the Dionysiac cult . . . 'left in the nature of Greek man a morbid inclination, a tendency to experience sudden and fleeting disturbances of his normal capacity to perceive and feel. Isolated pieces of information tell us of attacks of that transitory delirium, which affected whole cities in epidemic form.' Using present-day medical terminology rather broadly, it does not seem too venturesome to call the psychic life of the Greeks during their Middle Ages neurotic" (p. 40).

15. See Jeffrey Henderson, *The Maculate Muse,* p. 90. Henderson's work is invaluable in making clear the importance of obscene language to Old Comedy. The obscenities are not, as many people believe, an unfortunate remnant of primitive fertility cults. They are a deliberate component of an aggressive theater. As Henderson observes, "Clearly, the public enjoyed and demanded the presentation of obscenity in comedy; when the public largely ceased to do so, toward the end of the fifth century, comedy largely ceased to offer it" (p. 32).

16. Zeitlin, in "Cultic Models," writes that Athenians' "uneasiness about women in charge and women alone can be directly corroborated in . . . the *Thesmophoriazousae*" (p. 146).

17. "Psychomachia" as used in theater criticism need not be restricted to tableaus of virtue and vice. See Alan C. Dessen, *Elizabethan Drama and the Viewer's Eye,* p. 129, where Dessen defines the "stage psychomachia" as "a dramatic moment in which a figure about to make a significant decision is on stage with two or more figures who in some way act out the alternatives involved in that decision."

18. Mnesilochus's response to the servant's song is cruder than Rogers's "fudge" suggests, though *bombax* (45) and *bombalobombax* (48) are certainly difficult, if not impossible, to translate. Henderson describes ways in which sound effects were used in Old Comedy to signify crepitation or even a quasi-musical gurgling (p. 198). Mnesilochus is possibly imitating farting in order to indicate his disapproval of the performance, as the so-called Bronx cheer is often used for similar purposes—though these days without markedly obscene connotations.

19. Henderson, *The Maculate Muse,* p. 88.
20. Ibid., pp. 40, 153.
21. Rogers's note (pp. 140–41) is helpful on this point.
22. Henderson's translation (*The Maculate Muse,* p. 158).
23. See ibid., pp. 88–89.
24. Zeitlin, "Travesties," p. 196.
25. My translation.
26. Of Mnesilochus's transformation, Zeitlin writes, "The depilation of Mnesilochus is balanced by the putting on of women's clothing,

for in this ambivalent game of genders, the female is not only a 'not,' but also an 'other' " ("Travesties," p. 179).

27. See Rogers, p. 215, n. *b*.
28. See Henderson, *The Maculate Muse*, pp. 90–91.
29. On the general subject of the komos, see Adrados, *Festival, Comedy, Tragedy*, esp. pp. 37–49: "The *komos* from which Comedy derives is often understood as a festive procession of young people made merry with wine, sometimes disguised, sometimes involved in an erotic adventure. But this definition of the *komos*, in so far as it is correct, refers to a secondary, recent stage. The term *komos* at first had a wider meaning. It could refer to any of the various cortèges of choruses which performed a sacral action. These were the basis of all the theatrical genres, not Comedy alone. . . . Indeed, there are numerous testimonies to the fact that the term *komos* originally had a wider sense than that of a festal chorus of more or less comic type" (pp. 37–38).
30. Pickard-Cambridge in *Dithyramb, Tragedy, and Comedy* describes the initial entry of the chorus as an "invasion" that "rudely" interrupts the hero and his schemes (p. 212).
31. For a full discussion of the parabasis, see G. M. Sifakis, *Parabasis and Animal Choruses*. Sifakis argues that the parabasis of Old Comedy is not likely "a primitive element, a relic of a ritual embedded in the body of comedy. On the contrary, it is a sophisticated device which originated in the competitive spirit of the fifth century dramatic festivals, and developed in accordance with the rules of a dramatic technique that enabled the actors to address the audience either as characters of the play, or as members of a group of performers under the leadership of the poet-producer" (p. 68).
32. Goldman, *The Actor's Freedom*, pp. 55, 56.
33. Bennett Simon, *Mind and Madness in Ancient Greece*, p. 114.

2. The Comedy of Plautus

1. Eduard Fraenkel, *Plautinisches im Plautus*, esp. chap. 8 ("Die Vorherrschaft der Sklavenrolle"). A revised edition of Fraenkel's monumental study was published as *Elementi Plautini in Plauto*, trans. Franco Munari (Florence, 1960), but the work has never been translated into English, a great misfortune. Fraenkel's position is that Plautus *modified* existing slave roles; he cites "various opportunities to observe how much Plautus loves to expand the slave's role at the expense of other parts of the original" (*Es liess sich bereits bei verschiedenen Gelegenheiten beobachten, wie sehr Plautus es liebt, Sklavenrollen auf Kosten andere Bestandteile seiner Originale zu bereichern*, p. 240). A change of at least this magnitude seems certain, and

for my own purposes it does not matter whether or not Plautus can be said to have created the role ex nihilo, as is suggested by A. W. Gomme, in *Essays in Greek History and Literature,* p. 287.

2. Walter R. Chalmers, "Plautus and His Audience," p. 28.

3. Philippe E. Legrand, *The New Greek Comedy.* Legrande describes a mass influx of slaves in Latin comedy, a phenomenon which he attributes to a "certain Pharasaism on the part of the poets and of the spectators, to whom it was distasteful to represent or to see free men in positions that were unworthy of them. . . . It is the business of slaves to spare people who are so virtuous the annoyance of being compromised" (p. 217).

4. Cited in Segal, *Roman Laughter,* p. 140, and Chalmers, "Plautus and His Audience," p. 39.

5. See Turner, *The Ritual Process:* "The masking of the weak in aggressive strength and the concomitant masking of the strong in humility and passivity are devices that cleanse society of its structurally engendered 'sins'" (p. 185).

6. Segal, *Roman Laughter,* p. 141.

7. See Caputi, *Buffo.* Caputi writes: "I take vulgar comedy to be a creation, like the city, designed to make life more endurable, more secure, more enjoyable. Vulgar comedy, like its origins, embraces an intricate set of conventions for releasing within those experiencing it a sense that they have dominated all that opposes fruitfulness and health, an exhilaration which, even if only temporary, makes life tolerable" (pp. 93–94). The corollary to this view of comedy, of course, is that life is usually *not* tolerable. But we need not debate existential questions to object to seeing comic theater as no more significant than the cream in the coffee or the icing on the cake.

8. Northrop Frye, "The Argument of Comedy," p. 61. In a more recent study, *Roman Comedy,* David Konstan takes a similar view; of the typical romantic plot of New Comedy, for example, he writes, "The impulse that aspires to the forbidden is domesticated, gratified without danger to public conventions, and thus the threat to the city-state ideal of a closed conjugal group is averted. Conversely, the ideal itself is thereby affirmed" (pp. 24–25).

9. George E. Duckworth, *The Nature of Roman Comedy,* p. 290.

10. Orwell's essay is well known and is often anthologized. I cite from the *Collected Essays,* pp. 28–29.

11. See Charles Garton, *Personal Aspects of the Roman Theatre;* Garton suggests that Roman audiences were normally aware of characters as "enacted persons" and that "an actor's self was not obliterated by his roles. It was revealed, and was of interest, both apart from them and through them" (pp. 10, 31).

12. My text is *Epidicus,* trans. Paul Nixon, Loeb Classical Library edition, vol. 2. Unless otherwise noted, I quote from Nixon's translation.

13. See George E. Duckworth, ed., *T. MACCI PLAVTI: EPIDICVS,* pp. 97–98. Duckworth summarizes the arguments as to whether or not *Epidicus* ever included a prologue.

14. *Solus nunc es,* ("now you are alone").

15. *Quo in loco haec res sit vides, Epidice: nisi quid tibi in tete auxili est, absumptus es,* ("You see in what situation the matter is, Epidicus; unless you find some help within yourself, you are destroyed").

16. Duckworth, *EPIDICVS,* p. 154.

17. *Virgis dorsum despoliet meum,* ("lay waste to my back with a rod").

18. *Solve sane, si lubet,* ("loose me, if it pleases you").

19. *Age, si quid agis* (196; "Act, if you're going to act"). See Duckworth, *EPIDICVS,* p. 154.

20. For additional discussion of this point, see William E. Gruber, "The Wild Men of Comedy."

21. Hayden White, "The Forms of Wildness," p. 4.

22. *Vincere vis? em, ostendo manus; tu habes lora, ego te emere vidi. quid nunc cessas? colliga,* ("You wish to bind me? Here, I give you my hands. You have thongs, I saw you buy them. Why hesitate now? Bind me").

23. Brecht uses this example in discussing the purpose of "alienation effects"; *Brecht on Theatre,* p. 144.

24. For a discussion of empathy and the "mobile personality" as they figure in social development, see Daniel Lerner, *The Passing of Traditional Society,* pp. 43–54.

25. Chalmers's essay provides a brief summary of contemporary events and Roman theatrical development. See also W. Beare, *The Roman Stage,* and Tenney Frank, *Life and Literature in the Roman Republic,* esp. chaps. 1 ("Introduction: Social Forces") and 3 ("Greek Comedy on the Roman Stage").

26. Carl Kerényi, *The Religion of the Greeks and Romans,* p. 144.

27. Raymond Williams, *Modern Tragedy,* p. 30.

28. Goldman cites the choral ode from *Antigone* ("Wonders are many, but none more wondrous than man") and notes that "the word we translate as 'wondrous' can also mean 'strange' or 'terrifying' or even 'uncanny.'" He adds, "The Greek dramatic hero is always *deinos* in this sense" (p. 57).

29. The exact legal status of actors during this period is problematic. Cicero remarks (*De Re Publica,* IV.10) that all persons connected with the theater were denied their civic rights, but the reference is ambiguous. Epidicus seems to have been played in Plautus's time by Publilius Pellio, a Roman citizen (though possibly a freedman) and the actor-manager of a troupe (Garton, *Personal Aspects of the Roman Theatre,* p. 172). Clearly,

however, throughout the second century there was considerable opposition to the theater and to the actor's profession, which was considered disgraceful. See Frank, *Life and Literature*, pp. 95–98. The contrast with Athens, whose actors were esteemed, is striking and puzzling.

PART II. Renaissance Models

1. Greenblatt, Introduction, p. 5.
2. Wilson, "The Political Background of Shakespeare's *Richard II* and *Henry IV*," *Shakespeare-Jahrbuch* 75 (1939), cited by Greenblatt, p. 4.
3. Elizabeth's comment is well known; see the Arden edition of *Richard II*, pp. lvii–lxii.
4. Greenblatt, Introduction, p. 4.
5. Ibid., pp. 4, 3, and 4, respectively.
6. Hume, "English Drama and Theatre 1660–1800," p. 84.
7. Dollimore, *Radical Tragedy*, p. 28.
8. Kernan, *The Playwright as Magician*, p. 91.
9. Dollimore, *Radical Tragedy*, p. 4.
10. Moretti, "'A Huge Eclipse,'" pp. 7–8.
11. James K. Feibleman, "Critique of the Logic of Psychoanalysis." Feibleman writes: "By the historical fallacy is meant the definition of an entity in terms of its origins, the explanation of what a thing is by the description of how it came to be what it is" (p. 60).
12. But this important distinction has not always been observed. For a brief (and amusing) account of the abuses of myth criticism, see Patti P. Gillespie and Kenneth M. Cameron, *Western Theatre*, pp. 45–48.

3. Festive Comedy: *Bartholomew Fair*

1. Algernon Charles Swinburne, *A Study of Ben Jonson*, p. 60. But Swinburne added that the play belonged "among the minor and coarser masterpieces of comic art" (p. 62).
2. Thomas Greene, "Ben Jonson and the Centered Self," p. 346.
3. L. A. Beaurline, *Jonson and Elizabethan Comedy*, p. 254.
4. See C. L. Barber, *Shakespeare's Festive Comedy*, and his earlier essay, "Saturnalia in the Henriad."
5. See Douglas Duncan, *Ben Jonson and the Lucianic Tradition*, esp. pp. 1–6 and 203–12.
6. I borrow these terms from Timothy J. Wiles, *The Theater Event*, p. 4.
7. For a thorough discussion of the structure of *Bartholomew Fair*,

see Richard Levin, "The Structure of *Bartholomew Fair*" as well as his study *The Multiple Plot in English Renaissance Drama*, pp. 202–14.

8. See Freda L. Townsend, *Apologie for "Bartholomew Fayre,"* pp. 71–76.

9. According to Levin, *Bartholomew Fair* and Thomas Middleton's *A Chaste Maid in Cheapside* are so complex as to raise the question of "how much 'multiplicity' can be successfully integrated into a single dramatic whole" (*Multiple Plot*, p. 192).

10. "Bracket" follows Goffman's definition: the term denotes a conventional frame which walls off activity (especially recreational activity) from the rest of everyday life. See *Frame Analysis*, pp. 251–69.

11. I quote *Bartholomew Fair* from the Clarendon Press edition of Jonson's works; act, scene, and line numbers appear in my text.

12. On the psychology of bugging, see Goffman, *Frame Analysis*, pp. 156–200.

13. See Nicholas Grene, *Shakespeare, Jonson, Molière*, p. 9. Grene writes, "*Bartholomew Fair*, rather surprisingly, does not contain many opportunities for doubling except of very minor characters and extras" (p. 255). In this respect it is unique among Jonson's comedies. On early Elizabethan acting companies' practice of "doubling" roles to accommodate plays with many characters, see David Bevington, *From "Mankind" to Marlowe*, esp. pp. 104–13.

14. In *Shakespeare, Jonson, Molière*, Grene notes, "One of the peculiarities of *Bartholomew Fair*, and one which causes most trouble to readers, is the continuous thickening with new characters which we get right through the action. As late as IV.iv, we meet three characters we have never heard of before, Northern, Puppy and Cutting, and it does not help matters that we never hear of them again after this one scene. This is the point at which people reading the play who have been finding it hard to follow tend to give up in disgust" (p. 9). Keeping track of the characters is somewhat less difficult for a spectator, who has the actors' bodies and voices to help him remember identities, but the fact remains that in this play Jonson is assaulting his audience as never before.

15. See J. W. Binns, "'Women or Transvestites on the Elizabethan Stage?'" p. 96.

16. Beaurline, *Jonson and Elizabethan Comedy*, p. 253.

17. See Coburn Gum, *The Aristophanic Comedies of Ben Jonson;* the entire study is relevant.

18. Duncan, *Ben Jonson and the Lucianic Tradition*, p. 211.

19. T. S. Eliot, *The Sacred Wood*, p. 115.

20. See Kenneth Burke, *Counter-Statement;* Burke argues that "the psychology here [i.e., in *Hamlet*, I.iv.] is not the psychology of the *hero*, but the psychology of the *audience*. And by that distinction, form would

be the psychology of the audience. Or, seen from another angle, form is the creation of an appetite in the mind of the auditor, and the adequate satisfying of that appetite" (p. 31). Much of this part of my discussion of *Bartholomew Fair* borrows from Burke's reading of Hamlet's first encounter with his father's ghost.

21. Ibid., p. 124.
22. Ibid., p. 31.
23. Levin, *Multiple Plot,* p. 205.
24. See René Girard, "'To Entrap the Wisest,'" p. 117.
25. Beaurline, *Jonson and Elizabethan Comedy,* p. 4.
26. Ibid., p. 253.
27. Whether Jonson intends Winwife or Quarlous (or one of the pair) to guide the spectators' responses to *Bartholomew Fair* is a matter of much dispute. Levin (*Multiple Plot,* p. 214, n. 14) and Grene (*Shakespeare, Jonson, Molière,* p. 11) each provide a brief overview of debate on this point. Grene concedes that Quarlous and Winwife are the best of a bad lot, "the only characters with whom an audience could identify without damage to their self-respect" (p. 11). But he cautions against any wholehearted identification with them: "But all the same they scarcely fit the part of *raisonneurs* either singly or together. The analogy with the wits of *Epicoene* does not altogether hold. Truewit, Clerimont and Dauphine all have names which mark them quite clearly for the audience's approval, whereas Quarlous and Winwife have satiric-descriptive names which would suggest that they are to be viewed with the other comic characters" (p. 11).
28. Greene, "Ben Jonson and the Centered Self," p. 337.
29. See Stephen J. Greenblatt, *Renaissance Self-Fashioning;* the entire study is of considerable interest.
30. Greenblatt, "The False Ending in *Volpone,*" p. 104.

4. Shamming Illness and Shamming Identity:
Doctors and Actors in *Le malade imaginaire*

1. Frye, *Anatomy of Criticism,* p. 163.
2. Hubert, *Molière and the Comedy of Intellect,* p. 265. That Molière's own productions of *Le malade imaginaire* were played for laughter does not invalidate this point. Certainly, the spectators who assembled to see a new comedy by Molière would have expected the play and its chief actor to make them laugh. But the important matter is not whether or not onlookers laugh at Argan (or at Mnesilochus or Epidicus) but to what extremes, whether through laughter or tears, the actors' play leads them. On casting and its relationship to Molière's performance style, see Roger

W. Herzel, "Molière's Actors and the Question of Types"; "'Much Depends on the Acting'"; and *The Original Casting of Molière's Plays*.

3. My text is Molière, *Oeuvres complètes*, 2:1099–100. All quotations from *Le malade imaginaire* follow this edition; translations are mine.

4. See Seymour Chatman, *Story and Discourse*. Chatman writes that structuralist theory presupposes for every narrative a "content" and an "expression, the means by which the content is communicated" (p. 19).

5. That is, to what extent is a "plot summary" (such as the one I have just given) *itself* a "version" of the story? As any teacher of undergraduate courses in literature knows, the ability to summarize plots is not instinctive. It must be learned. It is illuminating, in this connection, to ask a child to summarize the "plot" of a familiar work. The child's abstracted version usually bears little resemblance to the myths scholars discuss with one another.

6. For an excellent discussion of contemporary antitheatricalism, see Henry Phillips, *The Theatre and Its Critics in Seventeenth Century France*. It is paradoxical, as Phillips observes, "that the century which saw the most brilliant single period of theatrical activity in French history, encouraged by the most powerful people in the land, should at the same time have been the target of a sustained and unrelenting attack from all quarters of the French Churches" (p. 3).

7. As to whether Argan's hypochondria is itself a manipulative ploy, I would distinguish between him and the rest of the characters on the basis of political motive. In the case of Toinette's playacting, the initiated observer can always see that appearances are being manipulated by a clever improviser; there is only one layer of deception, and a clear distinction is maintained between it and the real self that lies beneath it. Argan, however, manifests a more problematic relationship between appearances and reality. He *is* his humor; strip him of his imagined illness and nothing at all remains. See James F. Gaines, *Social Structures in Molière's Theater*, pp. 214–31. Gaines notes that, even in the final burlesque, "one wonders whether Argan is aware that he is masquerading" (p. 231, n. 30).

8. *Oeuvres* 2:1502; Herzel, *The Original Casting of Molière's Plays*, p. 83.

9. Gaines, *Social Structures in Molière's Theater*, p. 224.

10. On the specific subject of Molière's relationship with his doctors, see John Palmer, *Molière*, chap. 20 ("Impious in Medicine"). Palmer notes that during Molière's life "the dress and habit of the physician was still that of the sorcerer" (p. 416). On the subject of the doctor in Molière's comedy, see Grene, *Shakespeare, Jonson, Molière*, chap. 4 ("Quacks and Conmen"). I agree with Grene in that we need not imagine "a disturbed personal life feeding the life of the plays" (p. 81); but the response

to Molière/Argan is more problematic than Grene makes it seem, and it seems hardly possible to believe, as Grene does, that in *Le malade imaginaire* "the realities of pain and death, which must have been so very real to Molière by then, are tacitly ignored, while the audience can observe with uninfatuated amusement the infatuation of Argan and the 'gallimatias' of his doctors" (p. 82). See also Carlo François, "Médecine et religion chez Molière."

11. Herzel notes that this scene is the last ever played by Molière and his great colleague, La Grange. The scene, according to Herzel, "shows their on-stage relationship in its purest form, since it is almost independent of language: Argan and Purgon use words as talismans, and the magic of the incantation 'Monsieur Purgon!' cannot stand up against the magic of 'bradypepsie, dyspepsie, apepsie, lienterie, dysenterie, hydropisie, privation de la vie'" ("'Much Depends on the Acting,'" p. 356).

12. Luigi Pirandello, *Six Characters in Search of an Author;* all quoted statements appear on p. 265.

13. The last thing Toinette says to Argan is *tenez-vous bien.* Sometimes her comment is translated as "keep still," but it seems to me the situation is more tense than this idiom indicates. For Argan, the impending situation is supremely exciting; we must remember, after all, that he has never consciously playacted before. Toinette's words suggest the kind of remark we might make to a child about to embark on a first roller-coaster ride: "hang on tight" or something to that effect.

14. See Jacques Guicharnaud, introduction, p. 9.

15. Bertolt Brecht, *A Man's A Man,* 2:29. Brecht's German is impossible to translate without loss: *Mich kann man auch am Arsch lecken mit Charakterköpfen* ("One can lick my ass with character-heads" [portrait-studies]); *Gesammelte Werke* 1:329.

5. *The Cherry Orchard:* Text versus Performance

1. Chekhov's letters abound with the playwright's comments on his work. As the following excerpts from the letters make clear, Chekhov's sense of genre typically grew more acute as work on a play progressed.

To A. S. Souvorin
Moscow. Nov. 15, 1888.
Why do you refuse to write "The Demon of the Woods" in collaboration with me? If the play does not turn out well, or if you should dislike it, I give you my word not to produce it and not to publish it. If you do not like "The Demon" let us take some other subject. Let us write a tragedy, "Holofernes," on the motive of the opera "Judith," in which we shall make Judith love Holofernes; a good military leader slain through Jewish cunning. . . .

> *To A. S. Souvorin*
> Moscow. May 4, 1889.
> Imagine,—I am through with the first act of "The Demon of the Woods." The result is not so bad, though a bit long. I have greater confidence than when I wrote "Ivanov." The play will be completed by the beginning of June. . . . The play is very queer, and I wonder how this odd thing came from my pen. I am in dread as to the attitude of the Censor's office. . . .
>
> *To A. S. Souvorin*
> Luka. May 14, 1889.
> Shcheglov is not one of my competitors. I don't know his drama, but I feel that I accomplished ten times more in my first two acts than he in all his five acts. His play may have greater success than mine, but I do not dread such competition. I tell you this to show that I am satisfied with my work. The play is rather dull and something of a mosaic,—still it leaves upon me an impression of accomplishment. The characters have been entirely recast; there is no servant in the play, not one incidental figure for comic relief, not one widow. . . .
>
> *To A. N. Plescheyev*
> Moscow. Sept. 30, 1889.
> Imagine, I am writing a long comedy, and at a stretch I have written two and a half acts. After finishing a tale, one works on a comedy with ease. The characters are good, wholesome, and fairly likable people; and the ending is a happy one. The prevailing tone is crisp, lyric. The play is called "The Demon of the Woods." [*Letters on the Short Story, the Drama, and Other Literary Topics,* ed. Friedland, pp. 124–26]

Chekhov ultimately decided that his last work, *The Cherry Orchard,* was a comedy, and his dismay over Stanislavsky's production of this play has become legendary. On September 15, 1903, he described the play in a letter to Madame Stanislavsky: "It has turned out not a drama, but a comedy, in parts a farce" (ibid., p. 159). Chekhov did not attend the rehearsals for *The Cherry Orchard,* but he grew increasingly annoyed with the news that reached Yalta concerning the rehearsals and advance publicity for his play. He concluded that his play had been seriously distorted, and in ill health on October 23 he wrote to Vladimir Nemirovitch-Dantchenko to complain: "I don't know what to do, whether to go to Moscow or not. I'd very much like to sit in on some rehearsals and have a look at things. I'm afraid Anya will speak in a tearful tone of voice (for some reason you find her similar to Irina), I'm afraid she won't be played by a young actress. Anya never once cries in the play and nowhere does she even have tears in her voice. She may have tears in her eyes during the second act, but her tone of voice is gay and lively.

Why do you say in your telegram that there are many weepy people in my play? Where are they? Varya's the only one, and that's because she's a crybaby by nature. Her tears are not meant to make the spectator feel despondent. I often use "through her tears" in my stage directions, but that indicates only a character's mood, not actual tears. There's no cemetery in the second act" (*Letters of Anton Chekhov,* trans. Heim and Karlinsky, pp. 459–460).

2. Quoted in *Anton Chekhov's Plays,* p. 161. All quotations from *The Cherry Orchard* follow this work; page numbers in text refer to this edition. Chekhov believed that Stanislavsky had turned his comedy into a "drama," a term which at the time signified a specific kind of play. On April 10, 1904, Chekhov complained to Olga Knipper: "Why is it that on the posters and in the newspaper advertisements my play is so persistently called a drama? Nemirovitch and Stanislavsky see in my play something absolutely different from what I have written, and I am ready to bet anything that neither of them has once read my play through attentively. Forgive me, but I assure you it is so" (*The Letters of Anton Pavlovitch Tchehov to Olga Leonardovna Knipper,* trans. and ed. Garnett, p. 380).

3. For a summary of some performance traditions, see Siegfried Melchinger, "Stage Production in Europe," pp. 397–401. Melchinger describes a production of *The Three Sisters* at Prague's *Theatre Before the Gate* (1967) in which the silences constitute "a dismantling of the spoken words through that which happens behind, between, and beyond them" (p. 400). As for the sounds, they "thicken, jelling into surrealist music. The gestures, the walking, swing in its rhythm, and the constant play of movement and expression that underlies the dialogue becomes high-tension choreography" (p. 401).

4. We ought to heed the playwright's suggestion that we examine the text for performance values, as he was always telling Stanislavsky, although Stanislavsky apparently could not understand. Karlinsky observes that "a great deal of what is puzzling, paradoxical and nonsensical in the entire body of Chekhovian studies becomes clear and understandable the moment *My Life in Art* is removed from the scene as a basic source" (p. 394).

5. See E. H. Gombrich, *Art and Illusion,* esp. pp. 179–287 ("The Beholder's Share").

6. Robert Brustein, *The Theatre of Revolt,* pp. 168–69.

7. The concept "horizon of expectation" is borrowed from Hans-Robert Jauss, *Literaturgeschichte als Provokation,* pp. 175–76.

8. On January 4, 1889, Chekhov wrote to A. S. Souvorin: "You write that the stage lures you because it resembles life. . . . Is this so? But I think that the theatre lures you and me and shrivels Shcheglov up,

because it is a form of sport" (*Letters on the Short Story, the Drama, and Other Literary Topics*, p. 141). There is more involved here than a comparison of "good" and "bad" performances. Spectators' experience of theater involves an awareness of the tension between the players' activity and an exterior reality which constantly impinges upon it. An audience knows when the actors are succeeding and when their performance is for some reason too real or insufficient. See Donald M. Kaplan, "Gestures, Sensibilities, Scripts." Kaplan postulates "a sensibility very highly developed in humans, which discriminates between the animate and the inanimate" and which is essential to the experience of histrionic performance. In spectators, according to Kaplan, "this sensibility detects that the drive arousal (appetite) induced in the performer is being regulated by the gestures of a script rather than by the gestures of the performer's everyday life" (p. 32).

9. See Goldman, *The Actor's Freedom:* "Comedy of mechanism recalls Bergson, and it fits many comic effects well, but I see now that when we think about comic performance we are likely to find it a dangerous term. For in performance—at least when the performance is good—all comedy is the comedy of irrepressibility" (p. 89).

10. For example, W. S. Gilbert recommended a "realistic" playing style for his wildly improbable comedy *Engaged* (1877), a comedy of errors involving—in addition to the usual romantic confusions—salmon poachers, derailed trains, and border disputes. Yet Gilbert stressed, "It is absolutely essential to the success of this piece that it should be played with the most perfect earnestness and gravity throughout. There should be no exaggeration in costume, make-up, or demeanour; and the characters, one and all, should appear to believe, throughout, in the perfect sincerity of their words and actions. Directly the characters show that they are conscious of the absurdity of their utterances the piece begins to drag." Quoted in Michael Booth, *English Plays of the Nineteenth Century*, 3:330.

11. Audiences quickly learn to tune out most sounds which are not part of the performance; what Chekhov is doing is exploiting spectators' "disattend track." On the psychology of the "disattend track," see Goffman, *Frame Analysis*, pp. 220–23.

12. J. L. Styan, *Chekhov in Performance*, p. 253.

13. For a general discussion of the two possible modes of spectators' laughter, see Goffman, *Frame Analysis*, p. 130–31.

14. Charles B. Timmer, "The Bizarre Element in Čechov's Art," p. 278.

15. Styan, *Chekhov in Performance*, p. 337.

16. In his discussion of children's games and their evolution, Piaget describes a class of symbolic identifications open to elaborate develop-

ment: "These forms of play, which consist in liquidating a disagreeable situation by re-living it in make-believe, clearly illustrate the function of symbolic play, which is to assimilate reality to the ego while freeing the ego from the demands of accommodation. In the ordinary cases it is only a matter of intensifying the awareness of newly acquired powers, or of extending them through make-believe. In the case of type IIIB [games which involve correcting reality, not just its reproduction for pleasure] the ego is enabled to take its revenge on reality, *i.e.*, to compensate for it. In the case of type IIIC the proper function of the game is to reproduce in their entirety scenes in which the ego ran the risk of failure, thereby enabling it to assimilate them and emerge victorious. From the point of view of structure, then, there is exact imitation, but imitation with intent to subordinate the model imitated, and not to yield to it" (*Play, Dreams, and Imitation in Childhood*, p. 134). By constantly inviting the real world into his play, Chekhov demands that onlookers directly accommodate one to the other, an activity which the modern theatrical frame normally disallows.

17. There is an obvious comparison to be made here with the famous sound of a door being locked in *Ghosts*. Just before the end of Ibsen's tragedy, Osvald and his mother are briefly offstage:

> MRS. ALVING (*In the hall*) I must fetch a doctor, Osvald—let me out!
> OSVALD (*In the hall*) You shall not go out—and no one shall come in. (*Sound of a key turning in the lock*)
>
> [*Ghosts*, p. 90.]

The sound in *Ghosts* carries primarily thematic value; in *The Cherry Orchard*, however, it carries primarily closural value. The difference may be explained in terms of an audience's expectations. There is every reason to expect Osvald and his mother to reappear on stage, but in the mind of the audience the sudden appearance of Firs ironically falsifies the previous stage business: good-byes, sounds of locking doors, carriages driving off, and the dolorous chopping of the axes.

18. See Goldman, *The Actor's Freedom*, pp. 71–73.
19. *Meyerhold on Theatre*, pp. 32–33.

6. Comedy, Community, and the Anonymous Audience: Dürrenmatt's *Der Besuch der alten Dame*

1. The anecdote may be found in Paul Schwaber's essay "Freud and the Twenties."
2. See Jonas Barish, *The Antitheatrical Prejudice*. Barish traces throughout Western cultural history an abiding hostility to the theater

and theatrical behavior, a prejudice evident, for example, in expressions such as "don't make a scene."

3. My text is Friedrich Dürrenmatt, *Der Besuch der Alten Dame*, in *Komödien*, vol. 1. All quotations from *Der Besuch* (English translation: "The Visit") follow this edition; translations are mine.

4. Melvin Askew, "Dürrenmatt's *The Visit of the Old Lady*," p. 434.

5. Susanne Langer, *Feeling and Form*, pp. 355–56. Langer writes, "A dramatic act is a commitment. It creates a situation in which the agent or agents must necessarily make a further move; that is, it motivates a subsequent act (or acts)" (p. 355). I would add that a sensibility to this process of oppositional development is fundamental to the appreciation of drama. Consider, for example, the following (and possibly apocryphal) story that Nemirovitch-Dantchenko tells of Chekhov:

> In the editor's office of *Budilnik* the talk once turned on the benefits a writer received from being paid 'by the line,' and Chekhov argued that it was more profitable to write in short lines than in long periods, that it wouldn't do to imitate Gogol. He added that it was possible to receive as much for ten words as for ten solid lines.
>
> "Just try it!" said Kitcheyev, leaning back in his chair before the editorial table and playing with a long pencil.
> "And you'll pay?"
> "Yes, I'll pay."
>
> Chekhov remained standing for half a minute or so in a concentrated attitude, then snatched the pencil from Kitcheyev's hand and wrote on the spot.
>
> Dialogue
> "Listen!"
> "What?"
> "Native?"
> "Who?"
> "You."
> "I?"
> "Yes."
> "No."
> "Pity!"
> "H'm!"
>
> [*My Life in the Russian Theatre*, pp. 16–17]

This is not the place to attempt to discuss fully the reason that dramatic dialogue is "dramatic." My point is that both Dürrenmatt's and Chekhov's conversations develop by opposition and by inner necessity.

6. Askew, "Dürrenmatt's *The Visit of the Old Lady*," p. 436.

7. On the misunderstandings which have been perpetuated by blanket application of ritual models for dramatic action, see Richard F. Hardin, "'Ritual' in Recent Criticism." Among the many discussions of

The Visit, I have discovered none which devotes significant attention to the problems of text versus performance, which is where at least one area of interest surely lies.

    8. This is an enormous subject; I follow here the definition of the meaning of ritual action proposed by Mircea Eliade, *The Myth of the Eternal Return,* pp. 37–48. On the atemporal character of rite, see esp. chap. 2 ("The Regeneration of Time").

    9. Bergson writes: "Laughter is, above all, a corrective. Being intended to humiliate, it must make a painful impression on the person against whom it is directed. By laughter, society avenges itself for the liberties taken with it. It would fail in its object if it bore the stamp of sympathy or kindness" (*Laughter,* p. 187).

    10. Bergson, *Laughter,* p. 97.

    11. "Problems of the Theatre," p. 272.

    12. Dürrenmatt suggests that, to facilitate playing, Koby and Loby may speak alternately instead of together, omitting their characteristic echolalia (p. 358). To eliminate the repetitions, however, would by no means eliminate their oddly mechanical performance style.

    13. My reading here can be supplemented by E. S. Dick, "Dürrenmatt's *Der Besuch der alten Dame.*" Dick finds two separate orders of time represented in the play, one historical and one mythic, and argues (p. 506) that, in reconstructing Güllen, Dürrenmatt enacts the "raising" or the "annulment" of historical time (*die Aufhebung der Zeit*).

    14. Stanley Cavell, *Must We Mean What We Say?* p. 306.

    15. "Problems of the Theatre," p. 268.

Afterword: On Actors and Theatrical Genres

    1. Herbert Blau, *Take Up the Bodies,* p. 299.

    2. Nicolas Evreinoff, *The Theatre in Life,* p. 23.

    3. Blau, *Take Up the Bodies,* pp. 24–25.

    4. Goldman's entire book (*The Actor's Freedom*) bears on this point: "the leading role or roles of any play act out some version of a half-allowed, blasphemous, and sacred freedom characteristic of the era in which the play was written. In the enactment, by the very nature of the freedom pursued, the hero risks destruction" (p. 55).

    5. Kenneth Burke, *Dramatism and Development,* p. 29.

    6. *Brecht on Theatre,* p. 152.

Works Cited

Adrados, Francisco R. *Festival, Comedy, and Tragedy: The Greek Origins of Theatre*. Trans. Christopher Holme. Leiden: E. J. Brill, 1975.
Aristophanes, *Knights, Lysistrata,* and *Thesmophoriazusae*. In *Aristophanes*. Trans. B. B. Rogers. Loeb Classical Library. 1924. Rpt. Cambridge, Mass.: Harvard University Press, 1963.
Askew, Melvin. W. "Dürrenmatt's *The Visit of the Old Lady*." In *The Context and Craft of Drama*. Ed. Robert W. Corrigan and James L. Rosenberg. San Francisco: Chandler, 1964.
Bain, David. *Actors and Audience: A Study of Asides and Related Conventions in Greek Drama*. Oxford: Oxford University Press, 1977.
Barber, C. L. "Saturnalia in the Henriad." In *Shakespeare: Modern Essays in Criticism*. Ed. Leonard F. Dean. New York: Oxford University Press, 1961.
———. *Shakespeare's Festive Comedy: A Study of Dramatic Form and Its Relation to Social Custom*. Princeton: Princeton University Press, 1959.
Barish, Jonas. *The Antitheatrical Prejudice*. Berkeley: University of California Press, 1981.
Beare, W. *The Roman Stage: A Short History of Latin Drama in the Time of the Republic*. Cambridge, Mass.: Harvard University Press, 1951.
Beaurline, L. A. *Jonson and Elizabethan Comedy: Essays in Dramatic Rhetoric*. San Marino: Huntington Library, 1978.
Bergson, Henri. "Laughter." In *Comedy*. Introd. by Wylie Sypher. Garden City, N.Y.: Doubleday, Anchor Books, 1956.
Bevington, David. *From "Mankind" to Marlowe: Growth of Structure in the Popular Drama of Tudor England*. Cambridge, Mass.: Harvard University Press, 1962.
Binns, J. W. "'Women or Transvestites on the Elizabethan Stage?': An Oxford Controversy." *Sixteenth Century Journal* 5 (1974):95–120.
Blau, Herbert. *Take Up the Bodies: Theater at the Vanishing Point*. Urbana: University of Illinois Press, 1982.
Booth, Michael R. *English Plays of the Nineteenth Century*. Vol. 3: *Comedies*. Oxford: Clarendon Press, 1973.
Brecht, Bertolt. *Brecht on Theatre: The Development of an Aesthetic*. Ed. and trans. John Willett. New York: Hill and Wang, 1964.

———. *Collected Plays*, vol. 2. Ed. Ralph Manheim and John Willett. New York: Random House, 1977.
———. *Mann ist Mann*. In *Gesammelte Werke*, vol. 1. Frankfurt: Suhrkamp, 1967.
Brustein, Robert. *The Theatre of Revolt: An Approach to the Modern Drama*. Boston: Atlantic, Little, Brown, 1964.
Burke, Kenneth. *Counter-Statement*. 2d ed. Los Angeles: Hermes, 1953.
———. *Dramatism and Development*. Barre, Mass.: Clark University Press, 1972.
———. *The Philosophy of Literary Form: Studies in Symbolic Action*. Baton Rouge: Louisiana State University Press, 1941.
Caillois, Roger. *Man, Play, and Games*. Trans. Meyer Barash. New York: Crowell-Collier, 1961.
Caputi, Anthony. *Buffo: The Genius of Vulgar Comedy*. Detroit: Wayne State University Press, 1978.
Cavell, Stanley. *Must We Mean What We Say?* 1969. Rpt. Cambridge: Cambridge University Press, 1976.
Chalmers, Walter R. "Plautus and His Audience." In *Roman Drama*. Ed. T. A. Dorey and Donald R. Dudley. London: Routledge and Kegan Paul, 1965.
Chatman, Seymour. *Story and Discourse: Narrative Structure in Fiction and Film*. Ithaca: Cornell University Press, 1978.
Chekhov, Anton. *The Cherry Orchard*. In *Anton Chekhov's Plays*. Trans. and ed. Eugene K. Bristow. New York: Norton, 1977.
———. *Letters of Anton Chekhov*. Trans. Michael Henry Heim and Simon Karlinsky. Selection, commentary, and introduction by Simon Karlinsky. New York: Harper and Row, 1973.
———. *The Letters of Anton Pavlovitch Tchehov to Olga Leonardovna Knipper*. Trans. and ed. Constance Garnett. New ed. New York: Benjamin Blom, 1966.
———. *Letters on the Short Story, the Drama, and Other Literary Topics*. Ed. Louis S. Friedland. 1924. Rpt. New York: Benjamin Blom, 1964.
Cicero. *De Re Publica*. Trans. Clinton Walker Keyes. Loeb Classical Library.1928. Rpt.Cambridge, Mass.: Harvard University Press,1959.
Cornford, F. M. *The Origin of Attic Comedy*. London: E. Arnold, 1914.
Dessen, Alan C. *Elizabethan Drama and the Viewer's Eye*. Chapel Hill: University of North Carolina Press, 1977.
Dick, E. S. "Dürrenmatt's *Der Besuch der alten Dame:* Weltheater und Ritualspiel." *Zeitschrift für deutsche Philologie* 87 (1968):498–509.
Dollimore, Jonathan. *Radical Tragedy: Religion, Ideology, and Power in the Drama of Shakespeare and his Contemporaries*. Chicago: University of Chicago Press, 1984.

Duckworth, George. *The Nature of Roman Comedy: A Study in Popular Entertainment*. Princeton: Princeton University Press, 1952.
Duncan, Douglas. *Ben Jonson and the Lucianic Tradition*. Cambridge: Cambridge University Press, 1979.
Dürrenmatt, Friedrich. *Der Besuch der alten Dame*. In *Komödien*, vol. 1. Zurich: Peter Schifferli ["Die Arche"], 1957.
———. "Problems of the Theatre." Trans. Gerhard Nellhaus. In *The Context and Craft of Drama*. Ed. Robert W. Corrigan and James L. Rosenberg. San Francisco: Chandler, 1964.
Ehrmann, Jacques. "Homo Ludens Revisited." Trans. Cathy and Phil Lewis. In "Game, Play, Literature." *Yale French Studies* 41 (1968):31–57.
Eliade, Mircea. *The Myth of the Eternal Return*. Trans. Willard R. Trask. Bollingen Series, 46. 1954. Rpt. Princeton: Princeton University Press, 1974.
Eliot, T. S. *The Sacred Wood: Essays on Poetry and Criticism*. 6th ed. London: Methuen, 1948.
Evreinoff, Nicolas. *The Theatre in Life*. Ed. and trans. Alexander I. Nazaroff. 1927. Rpt. New York: Benjamin Blom, 1970.
Feibleman, James K. "Critique of the Logic of Psychoanalysis." *International Journal of Individual Psychology* 2 (1936):55–65.
———. *In Praise of Comedy: A Study in Its Theory and Practice*. New York: Horizon Press, 1970.
Fergusson, Francis. *The Idea of a Theater*. 1949. Rpt. Princeton: Princeton University Press, 1968.
Fowler, Alastair. *Kinds of Literature: An Introduction to the Theory of Genres and Modes*. Cambridge, Mass.: Harvard University Press, 1982.
Fraenkel. Eduard. *Plautinisches im Plautus*. Berlin: Weidmannsche Buchhandlung, 1922.
François, Carlo. "Médecine et religion chez Molière: Deux facettes d'une même absurdité." *French Review* 42 (1969):665–72.
Frank, Tenney. *Life and Literature in the Roman Republic*. Berkeley: University of California Press, 1930.
Frye, Northrop. *Anatomy of Criticism: Four Essays*. Princeton: Princeton University Press, 1957.
———. "The Argument of Comedy." In *English Institute Essays, 1948*. Ed. D. A. Robertson, Jr. New York: Columbia University Press, 1949.
Gaines, James F. *Social Structures in Molière's Theater*. Columbus: Ohio State University Press, 1984.
Garton, Charles. *Personal Aspects of the Roman Theatre*. Toronto: A. M. Hakkert, 1972.

Gillespie, Patti P., and Kenneth M. Cameron. *Western Theatre: Revolution and Revival.* New York: Macmillan, 1984.

Girard, René. "'To Entrap the Wisest': A Reading of *The Merchant of Venice.*" In *Literature and Society: Selected Papers from the English Institute,* n.s. 3. Ed. Edward W. Said. Baltimore: Johns Hopkins University Press, 1980.

Goffman, Erving. *Frame Analysis: An Essay on the Organization of Experience.* Cambridge, Mass.: Harvard University Press, 1974.

Goldman, Michael. *The Actor's Freedom: Toward a Theory of Drama.* New York: Viking Press, 1975.

Gombrich, E. H. *Art and Illusion: A Study in the Psychology of Pictorial Representation.* Bollingen Series 35. New York: Pantheon, 1960.

Gomme, A. W. *Essays in Greek History and Literature.* Oxford: Basil Blackwell, 1937.

Greenblatt, Stephen J. "The False Ending in *Volpone.*" *JEGP* 75 (1976):90–104.

———. Introduction to *The Power of Forms in the English Renaissance.* Ed. Stephen J. Greenblatt. Norman, Okla.: Pilgrim Books, 1982.

———. *Renaissance Self-Fashioning: From More to Shakespeare.* Chicago: University of Chicago Press, 1980.

Greene, Thomas. "Ben Jonson and the Centered Self." *SEL* 10 (1970): 325–48.

Grene, Nicholas. *Shakespeare, Jonson, Molière: The Comic Contract.* Totowa, N.J.: Barnes and Noble, 1980.

Gruber, William E. "The Polarization of Tragedy and Comedy." *Genre* 13 (1980):259–74.

———. "Systematized Delirium: The Craft, Form, and Meaning of Aristophanic Comedy." *Helios,* n.s. 10 (1983):97–111.

———. "The Wild Men of Comedy: Transformations in the Comic Hero from Aristophanes to Pirandello." *Genre* 14 (1981):207–27.

Guicharnaud, Jacques. Introduction to *Molière: A Collection of Critical Essays.* Englewood Cliffs, N.J.: Prentice-Hall, 1964.

Gum, Coburn. *The Aristophanic Comedies of Ben Jonson: A Comparative Study of Jonson and Aristophanes.* The Hague: Mouton, 1969.

Gurewitch, Morton. *Comedy: The Irrational Vision.* Ithaca: Cornell University Press, 1975.

Hardin, Richard F. "'Ritual' in Recent Criticism: The Elusive Sense of Community." *PMLA* 98 (1983):846–62.

Henderson, Jeffrey. *The Maculate Muse: Obscene Language in Attic Comedy.* New Haven: Yale University Press, 1975.

Herzel, Roger W. "Molière's Actors and the Question of Types." *Theatre Survey* 16 (1975):1–24.

———. "'Much Depends on the Acting': The Original Cast of *Le misanthrope.*" *PMLA* 95 (1980):348–66.
———. *The Original Casting of Molière's Plays.* Ann Arbor: UMI Research Press, 1981.
Howard, Jean E. "Figures and Grounds: Shakespeare's Control of Audience Perception and Response." *SEL* 20 (1980):185–99.
Hubert, J. D. *Molière and the Comedy of Intellect.* Berkeley: University of California Press, 1962.
Huizinga, Johan. *Homo Ludens: A Study of the Play Element in Culture.* 1949. Rpt. Boston: Beacon, 1955.
Hume, Robert D. "English Drama and Theatre, 1660–1800: New Directions in Research." *Theatre Survey* 23 (1982):71–100.
Ibsen, Henrik. *Ghosts.* Trans. Eva LeGallienne. In *Masters of Modern Drama.* Ed. Haskell M. Block and Robert G. Shedd. New York: Random House, 1962.
Jauss, Hans-Robert. *Literaturgeschichte als Provokation.* Frankfurt: Suhrkamp, 1970.
Jonson, Ben. *Ben Jonson.* Ed. C. H. Herford, Percy Simpson, and Evelyn Simpson. Oxford: Clarendon Press, 1938.
Kaplan, Donald M. "Gestures, Sensibilities, Scripts: Further Reflections on Performance/Audience Interactions." *Performance* 1 (1971):31–46.
Kerényi, C. *The Religion of the Greeks and Romans.* Trans. Christopher Holme. London: Thames and Hudson, 1962.
Kernan, Alvin B. *The Playwright as Magician: Shakespeare's Image of the Poet in the English Public Theater.* New Haven: Yale University Press, 1979.
Konstan, David. *Roman Comedy.* Ithaca: Cornell University Press, 1983.
Laín Entralgo, Pedro. *The Therapy of the Word in Classical Antiquity.* Ed. and trans. L. J. Rather and John M. Sharp. New Haven: Yale University Press, 1970.
Langer, Susanne. *Feeling and Form: A Theory of Art.* New York: Charles Scribner's Sons, 1953.
Legrand, Philippe E. *The New Greek Comedy.* Trans. James Loeb. 1917. Rpt. Westport, Conn.: Greenwood Press, 1970.
Lerner, Daniel. *The Passing of Traditional Society: Modernizing the Middle East.* Glencoe, Ill.: Free Press, 1958.
Levin, Richard. *The Multiple Plot in English Renaissance Drama.* Chicago: University of Chicago Press, 1971.
———. "The Structure of *Bartholomew Fair.*" *PMLA* 80 (1965):172–79.
Maus, Katharine Eisaman. "'Playhouse Flesh and Blood': Sexual Ideology and the Restoration Actress." *ELH* 46 (1979):595–617.

Melchinger, Siegfried. "Stage Productions in Europe." In *Anton Chekhov's Plays*. Trans. and ed. Eugene K. Bristow. New York: Norton, 1977.
Meyerhold, Vsevolod. *Meyerhold on Theatre*. Trans. and ed. Edward Braun. New York: Hill and Wang, 1969.
Molière. *Oeuvres complètes*. Ed. Georges Couton. Paris: Editions Gallimard, 1971.
Moretti, Franco. "'A Huge Eclipse': Tragic Form and the Deconsecration of Sovereignty." In *The Power of Forms in the English Renaissance*. Ed. Stephen Greenblatt. Norman, Okla.: Pilgrim Books, 1982.
Nagler, A. M. *A Source Book in Theatrical History*. 1952. Rpt. New York: Dover, 1959.
Nemirovitch-Dantchenko, Vladimir. *My Life in the Russian Theatre*. Trans. John Cournos. 1936. Rpt. London: Geoffry Bles, 1968.
Orwell, George. "Marrakech." In *Collected Essays*. London: Secker and Warburg, 1961.
Palmer, John. *Molière*. New York: Brewer and Warren, 1930.
Pavis, Patrice. *Languages of the Stage: Essays in the Semiology of the Theatre*. New York: Performing Arts Journal Publications, 1982.
Phillips, Henry. *The Theatre and Its Critics in Seventeenth Century France*. London: Oxford University Press, 1980.
Piaget, Jean. *Play, Dreams, and Imitation in Childhood*. Trans. C. Gattegno and F. M. Hodgson. New York: Norton, 1962.
Pickard-Cambridge, Sir Arthur. *Dithyramb, Tragedy, and Comedy*. 2d ed. rev. T. B. L. Webster. Oxford: Clarendon Press, 1962.
Pirandello, Luigi. *Six Characters in Search of an Author*. English version by Edward Storer. In *Naked Masks: Five Plays by Luigi Pirandello*. Ed. Eric Bentley. New York: E. P. Dutton, 1952.
Plautus. *Epidicus*. Trans. Paul Nixon. Loeb Classical Library. Vol. 2. 1917. Rpt. Cambridge, Mass.: Harvard University Press, 1977.
———. *T. MACCI PLAVTI: EPIDICVS*. Ed. George Duckworth. Princeton: Princeton University Press, 1940.
Rau, Peter. *Paratragodia: Untersuchung einer komischen Form des Aristophanes*. Munich: C. H. Beck, 1967.
Schwaber, Paul. "Freud and the Twenties." *Massachusetts Review* 22 (1981):133–51.
Schwartzman, Helen B. *Transformations: The Anthropology of Children's Play*. New York: Plenum Press, 1978.
Segal, Erich. *Roman Laughter: The Comedy of Plautus*. Cambridge, Mass.: Harvard University Press, 1968.
Shakespeare. *The Merchant of Venice*. Ed. John Russell Brown. Arden ed. 1955. Rpt. New York: Random House, 1964.

———. *Richard II.* Ed. Peter Ure. Arden ed. Cambridge, Mass.: Harvard University Press, 1956.
———. *The Tempest.* Arden ed. Ed. Frank Kermode. 1958. Rpt. London: Methuen, 1966.
Sifakis, G. M. *Parabasis and Animal Choruses: A Contribution to the History of Attic Comedy.* London: Athlone Press, 1971.
Simon, Bennett. *Mind and Madness in Ancient Greece: The Classical Roots of Modern Psychiatry.* Ithaca: Cornell University Press, 1978.
Stevens, Phillips, Jr., ed. *Studies in the Anthropology of Play: Papers in Memory of B. Allan Tindall.* West Point, N.Y.: Leisure Press, 1977.
Styan, J. L. "Changeable Taffeta: Shakespeare's Characters in Performance." In *Shakespeare: The Theatrical Dimension.* Ed. Philip C. McGuire and David A. Samuelson. New York: AMS Press, 1979.
———. *Chekhov in Performance: A Commentary on the Major Plays.* London: Cambridge University Press, 1971.
Swinburne, Algernon Charles. *A Study of Ben Jonson.* London: Chatto and Windus, 1889.
Timmer, Charles B. "The Bizarre Element in Čechov's Art." In *Anton Čechov, 1860–1960.* Ed. T. Eekman. Leiden: E. J. Brill, 1960.
Townsend, Freda L. *Apologie for "Bartholmew Fayre": The Art of Jonson's Comedies.* New York: Modern Language Association, 1947.
Turner, Victor. *Dramas, Fields, and Metaphors: Symbolic Action in Human Society.* Ithaca: Cornell University Press, 1974.
———. *The Ritual Process: Structure and Anti-Structure.* Chicago: Aldine, 1969.
Wagner, Roy. *Habu: The Innovation of Meaning in Daribi Religion.* Chicago: University of Chicago Press, 1972.
White, Hayden. "The Forms of Wildness: Archaeology of an Idea." In *The Wild Man Within: An Image in Western Thought from the Renaissance to Romanticism.* Ed. Edward Dudley and Maximillian E. Novak. Pittsburgh: University of Pittsburgh Press, 1972.
Whitman, Cedric H. *Aristophanes and the Comic Hero.* Cambridge, Mass.: Harvard University Press, 1964.
Wiles, Timothy J. *The Theater Event: Modern Theories of Performance.* Chicago: University of Chicago Press, 1980.
Williams, Raymond. *Modern Tragedy.* Stanford: Stanford University Press, 1966.
Zeitlin, Froma I. "Cultic Models of the Female: Rites of Dionysus and Demeter." *Arethusa* 15 (1982):129–57.
———. "Travesties of Gender and Genre in Aristophanes' *Thesmophoriazusae.*" In *Reflections of Women in Antiquity.* Ed. Helene P. Foley. New York: Gordon and Breach, 1981.

Index

Absurdist theater, 146–47
Acting style, 7, 18, 43–44, 49–52, 101, 127, 129
Actor-audience relationship: definition, 2, 7–8; in Old Comedy, 11, 19, 37; in Plautine comedy, 50–51, 55–58; in *Bartholomew Fair*, 74, 80–82, 88; in *Le malade imaginaire*, 118; in the modern period, 124; in Chekhov, 127, 136, 139; in Dürrenmatt, 161–63
Actor-character relationship: defined, 1–6; in Old Comedy, 17–19; in Plautus, 49–52; in Molière, 101; in Chekhov, 127, 132–34, 136; in Dürrenmatt, 157. *See also* Figur, Person-role formula
Aeschylus, 22
Agon, 38; dramatized, 90
Alazon, 17, 24
Alienation effect, 51, 175 (n. 23)
Antitheatricalism: Roman, 63, 65, 175 (n. 29); Tudor and Stuart, 77–80, 91; in seventeenth-century France, 105, 116, 118, 179 (n. 6); modern, 148, 163, 184–85 (n. 2)
Aristophanes, 11–41, 64, 78, 93, 129, 144; *Lysistrata*, 3, 4, 6, 14; *Frogs*, 12; *Ecclesiazusae*, 14; *Thesmophoriazusae*, 14, 19–41, 45; *Acharnians*, 14–19, 28, 62; *Birds*, 38; *Peace*, 38; *Wasps*, 38, 39; *Plutus*, 41, 61. *See also* Old Comedy
Aristotle, 2, 44, 52, 168
Askew, Melvin, 151, 153

Assimilation: as mimetic strategy, 14, 19, 28, 58–60, 63; as cultural adaptation, 63–64

Bacon, Francis, 80
Bain, David, 18
Barry, Elizabeth, 2, 3
Beaurline, L. A., 71, 78, 91–92
Beauval, Louise, 107
Bergson, Henri, 2, 118, 149, 156
Blau, Herbert, 166–67
Blocking character, 105
Bomolochos, 24, 34, 157, 162
Boucicault, Dion, 128
Bracket, 8, 73, 96–97, 132
Brecht, Bertolt, 7, 168; *Mann ist Mann*, 121–22, 127
Brustein, Robert, 128
Buffo. *See* vulgar comedy
Bulwer-Lytton, Edward, 123
Burke, Kenneth, 6, 84, 167

Cambridge anthopologists, 13
Caputi, Anthony, 43
Catharsis, 6, 19, 37, 43, 48, 60, 110, 137; in seventeenth-century medical theory, 102–3
Cavell, Stanley, 160
Chalmers, Walter, 43
Chekhov, Anton: *The Cherry Orchard*, 6, 125–45, 159; *The Sea Gull*, 125; *Three Sisters*, 125; *Uncle Vanya*, 144
Cleon (Athenian demagogue), 16–17
Colman, George (elder and younger), 123
Comic tradition, 6, 41, 61–63, 67, 70, 100–101, 104–5, 123
Cornford, F. M., 13

Darwinism (model for literary tradition), 123
Derrida, Jacques, 1
Disattend track, 59, 183 (n. 11)
Dollimore, Jonathan, 69–70
Dramatic illusion, 13, 16, 18, 142
Duckworth, George, 44
Duncan, Douglas, 82
Dürrenmatt, Friedrich: *Der Besuch der alten Dame*, 6, 145, 146–63; "Problems of the Theatre," 146, 156, 162

Eiron, 17
Eliot, T. S., 83–84
Elizabeth I, 68–69
Emerson, Ralph Waldo, 123
Empathy, 28–29, 63, 93, 134, 148; as transgression, 117; Brecht's objection to, 168. *See also* Identification.
English Civil War, 69–70
Essex rebellion, 68–69
Euripides, 14, 17, 21, 26–27, 34; *Telephus*, 14, 16; characterized in Aristophanic comedy, 14–18, 20–36, passim; *The Bacchae*, 26–27, 29, 32, 40–41
Evreinoff, Nicolas, 166
Excommunication: of actors, 105; ritual of, 112

Farce, 119, 128–31, 144, 157
Feibleman, James, 70, 165
Fergusson, Francis, 67
Festive comedy, 43, 64, 71–74, 82, 90–92, 98–99. *See also* Inversion ritual, Misrule, Status reversal
Festive frame, 73–74
Figur, 1, 8, 44, 46, 53, 55, 65, 133, 147. *See also* Actor-character relationship, Person-role formula
Fraenkel, Eduard, 42
Frame: play frame, 14, 22, 32, 36, 54–55, 148; as mode of cognition, 19–20; primary frame, 45, 64; recreational frame, 73–74, 82; representational (realistic) frame, 133–34, 148, 161; errors in framing, 158. *See also* Festive frame, Theatrical frame
Freud, Sigmund, 46, 149
Frye, Northrop, 43, 101

Gaines, James, 107, 179 (n. 7)
Gestus, Grundgestus: definitions, 7; in Old Comedy, 17, 22, 28, 32, 39; in Plautus, 51, 53, 59; in *Bartholomew Fair*, 77, 98–99; in *Le malade imaginaire*, 101, 109, 113, 118–119, 122; in Chekhov, 127, 129–30, 135–36, 139, 143; in Dürrenmatt, 161
Goffman, Erving, 8, 45
Goldman, Michael, 39
Gombrich, E. H., 127
Greenblatt, Stephen, 68, 99
Greene, Thomas, 71, 94
Grotowski, Jerzy, 148

Hazlitt, William, 4
Henderson, Jeffrey, 24–25
Historical fallacy, 70, 176 (n. 11)
Histrionic force, 7, 45, 52, 77, 105, 130–31, 134, 159
Hope Theatre, 71
Horizon of expectations, 128, 144
Hubert, J. D., 101
Hume, Robert, 69
Humors comedy, 62, 100, 130–31

Identification, 17–19, 28–29, 32, 45–46, 53–56, 59–60, 63, 79, 88–91, 93–94, 167–68, 179 (n. 27). *See also* empathy
Identity formation, 58–59, 119; relationship to acting, 167–68. *See also* Self
Imitation, 8, 28, 59, 167–68. *See also* Mimesis
Inversion ritual, 43, 45–46, 49, 56–58, 60, 70–74. *See also* Festive comedy, Misrule, Status reversal
Irving, Henry, 4, 5

James I, 95, 97–98
Jansenism, 122
The Jew of Venice, 4
Jonson, Ben, 123–24; *Bartholomew Fair*, 6, 62, 71–99, 130–31; *Volpone*, 94–95, 99; *The Alchemist*, 96; *Epicoene*, 96; *Every Man in his Humour*, 96

Kaprow, Allan, 148
Kean, Edmund, 4, 5
Kerényi, Carl, 64
Kernan, Alvin, 67
Komos, 38, 173 (n.29)

Lambard, William, 68
Langer, Susanne, 165
Legrand, Philippe, 43
Levin, Richard, 72
Link monologue, 50, 54
Lord Chamberlain's Men, 68
Louis XIII, 105
Lucianic satire, 72

Macklin, Charles, 4–5
Madness, 31, 78, 90, 114
Mannered comedy, 123
Maugham, Somerset, 123
Maus, Katherine, 2–3
Melodrama, 128
Menander, 101, 123
Meyerhold, Vsevolod, 143–44, 165
Mimesis: as critical term, 2, 19; Platonic views on, 29, 46; in New Comedy, 50, 52. *See also* Imitation
Misrule, 43, 45–46, 49, 56–58, 60, 70–74, 98–99. *See also* Festive comedy, Inversion ritual, Status reversal
Molière, 124; *Le malade imaginaire*, 6, 62, 100–122; *L'avare*, 100; *Le misanthrope*, 100; *Tartuffe*, 100; *Le médecin malgré lui*, 119, 121
Mommsen, Theodore, 43
Monitoring, 21, 54, 75, 79, 82, 92, 161. *See also* Seeing
Moretti, Franco, 70

Moscow Art Theatre, 125, 143
Mythos (of comedy), 98, 101, 105, 109, 118

New Comedy, 41, 42–65, 100–101, 103–5, 118, 123. *See also* Molière, Plautus
New critics, 68–69
New historicism, 68–70
"New society" of comedy, 57, 104–5

Obscene language, 13, 24–25; as defense mechanism, 27; as mode of aggression, 30–35; and tendency wit, 89
Old Comedy, 3–4, 11–41, 51, 59, 64, 78–79. *See also* Aristophanes
Okholopov, Nikolai, 148
Orwell, George, 44–45

Parabasis, 13, 16, 38–39, 173 (n. 31)
Parados, 38
Performance style: definition, 7; of Old Comedy, 17–19; in Plautus, 49–52; Chekhovian styles, 125, 128–31, 182 (n. 3); in Dürrenmatt, 156–57, 159–60
Person-role formula, 49, 101, 105. *See also* Actor-character relationship, Figur
Piaget, Jean, 8, 142
Pinero, Arthur Wing, 123
Pinter, Harold, 121, 123, 127
Pirandello, Luigi, 118–19
Plato, 31, 104
Plautus, 6, 42–65, 93, 105, 123, 129; *Epidicus*, 6, 41, 47–70; *Cistellaria*, 42; *Mercator*, 42; *Menaechmi*, 42, 47; *Amphitruo*, 47; *Bacchidae*, 47. *See also* New Comedy
Play within the play, 17–19, 20–24, 27–28, 30, 37, 47–61 passim, 82–92 passim, 104, 106, 108, 120
Punic Wars, 63

Reader-response criticism, 8
Realism: in Plautus, 43–44, 50–52; in Molière, 108; in Chekhov, 127–28, 132, 134, 139–40
Recreational frame. *See* Festive frame
Reinhardt, Max, 4
Ritual, 13–14, 17, 20, 67, 72, 134, 151, 153–54, 159–60, 163, 173 (n. 31); ritual action defined, 153–54; misapplication of ritual models to drama, 185 (n. 7)

Satire, 57, 72, 79–80, 103
Scapegoats and scapegoating, 28, 35, 115, 149, 160, 167
Schadenfreude, 46, 149
Schechner, Richard, 148
Scriptings and scripted responses, 8, 39, 55, 75–76, 89, 93, 97; awareness of scripts, 109, 129, 131; illusion of "scriptedness," 134, 182–83 (n. 8)
Seeing, 20, 24, 32, 44–45; forbidden seeing, 20, 27, 40, 64; precursor to identification, 27, 29; as understanding, 27–28, 60, 64; relationship to sexuality, 29, 40; and theatrical frame, 52; contrasted with observing, 74–75; moral implications of, 74–75, 79–80, 91–92. *See also* Monitoring
Segal, Erich, 43
Self: self-representing in Old Comedy, 18–19; self- invention in Plautus, 45, 52–53, 57–61; truth to self, 105, 109, 113–14; real vs. role, 117; self-definition, 117–19; selflessness, 118; exterior models for, 121
Senex, 128
Shakespeare: *The Winter's Tale*, 1, 108; *The Merchant of Venice*, 4, 5; *Richard II*, 68–69; *Love's Labor's Lost*, 83; *A Midsummer Night's Dream*, 83, 86; *Hamlet*, 84–85; *The Tempest*, 122

Shylock (transformations of the role), 4–5
Sidney, Philip, 87
Simon, Bennett, 40
Smithfield Fair, 72–74
Socrates (*Symposium*), 146
Sophocles, 149
Souvorin, A. S., 125, 180–81 (n. 1)
Sparagmos, 117
Stanislavsky, Konstantin, 125, 143
Status reversal, 43, 45–46, 49, 56–58, 60, 70, 72. *See also* Festive comedy, Inversion ritual, Misrule
Styan, J. L., 5, 136, 140, 143
Stychomythia, 153
Swinburne, Algernon, 71

Tate, Nahum, 2
Terence, 101
Text vs. performance, 2, 157; in *The Cherry Orchard*, 125–45
Theatrical frame, 18, 27, 52, 55, 60, 76–77, 80, 86, 96–97, 99, 118, 127, 131–32, 147–48, 159–61, 183–84 (n. 16)
Therapy (and theater), 35–37, 40, 43, 57–60, 101–3, 106, 109–14, 120, 134
Timmer, Charles, 140
Tragedy, 19, 25, 27, 40, 67, 70, 144, 146–47, 151, 153, 163, 167, 171 (n. 8)
Tragicomedy, 134, 147
Transvestite acting, 1, 3, 4; relationship to patriarchal audience, 3, 4, 20–41 passim; Deuteronomic injunction against, 77–78

Vulgar comedy, 43

White, Hayden, 56–57
Williams, Raymond, 64
Wilson, J. Dover, 68–69

Zeitlin, Froma, 19–20, 26–27

OHIO UNIVERSITY LIBRARY

Please return this book as soon as you have finished with it. In order to avoid a fine it must be returned by the latest date stamped below.

FEB 1 1 1994
QUARTER LOAN
AUG 2 4 1987   MAR 2 7 1995

QUARTER LOAN
JAN 4 1988   DEC 0 2 2005
RETURN BY   RECEIVED
            JUL 0 7 2008
MAY 3 1 1988

NOV 3 0
JUN 1 1988
    NON UNIV.

    1 5 199

RECEIVED
NOV 2 2 2005
DEC 0 4 2006

SEP 1 2 1986